HISTORY OF MEDICINE

L. Hartley

GENERAL EDITOR Jon Nichol

Contents

STANLEY THORNES

Introduction

When historians write the history of medicine they look at the evidence the past has left behind. For most periods of time the historian can consult many different kinds of evidence like these:

Pictorial/Visual	**Written**	**Artefacts**
Prints	Books	Tools
Drawings	Diaries	Pottery
Paintings	Letters	Coins
Photographs	Stone tablets	Statues
Maps		

A The title page of the 1588 edition of the works of the Greek doctor, Hippocrates

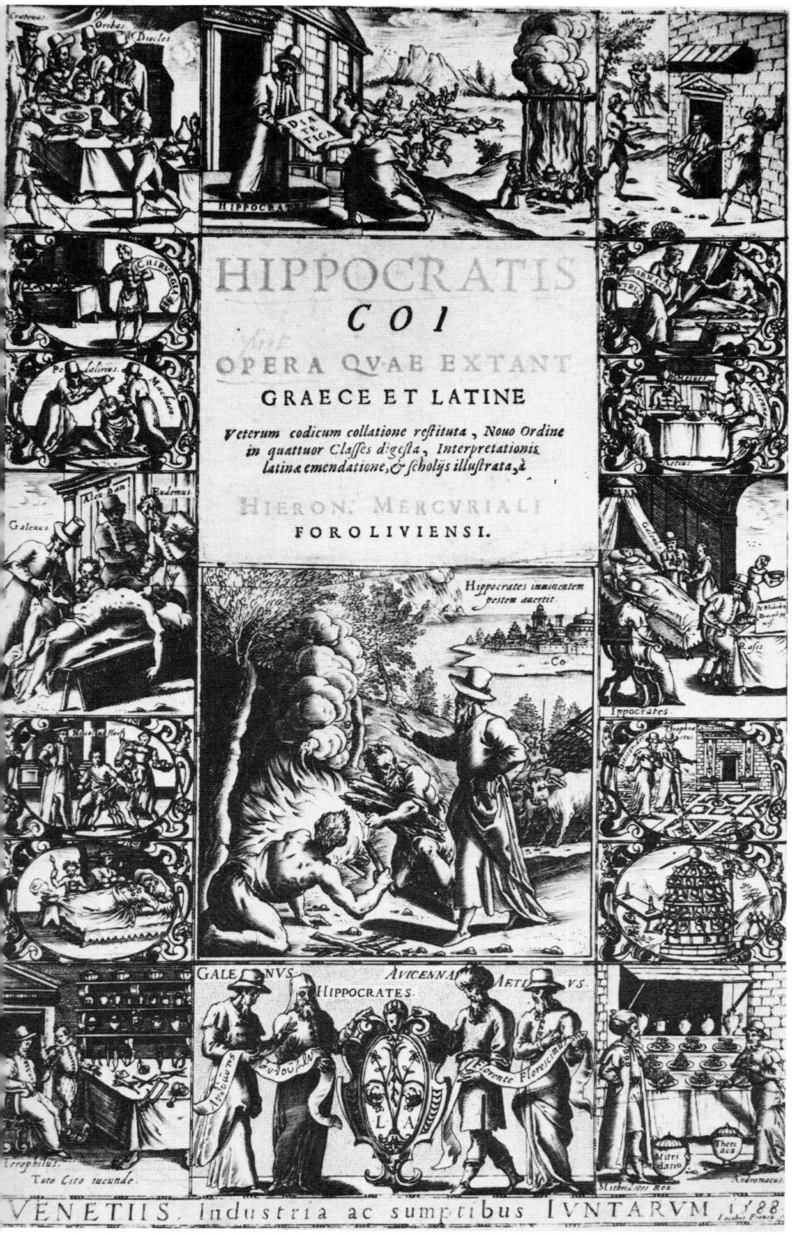

HIPPOCRATIS
COI
OPERA QVAE EXTANT
GRAECE ET LATINE
Veterum codicum collatione restituta, Nouo Ordine in quattuor Classes digesta, Interpretationis latinae emendatione, & scholijs illustrata, à
HIERON. MERCVRIALI
FOROLIVIENSI.
VENETIIS, industria ac sumptibus IVNTARVM 1588

Some evidence is primary evidence. This means it comes from the period of time the historian is studying. So, it could be a bone from prehistoric times like **B** or a nineteenth-century invention like **C**. Secondary evidence comes from a period of time later than the one that is being studied. This book is secondary evidence because, although it is about medicine in the past, it was written in 1983.

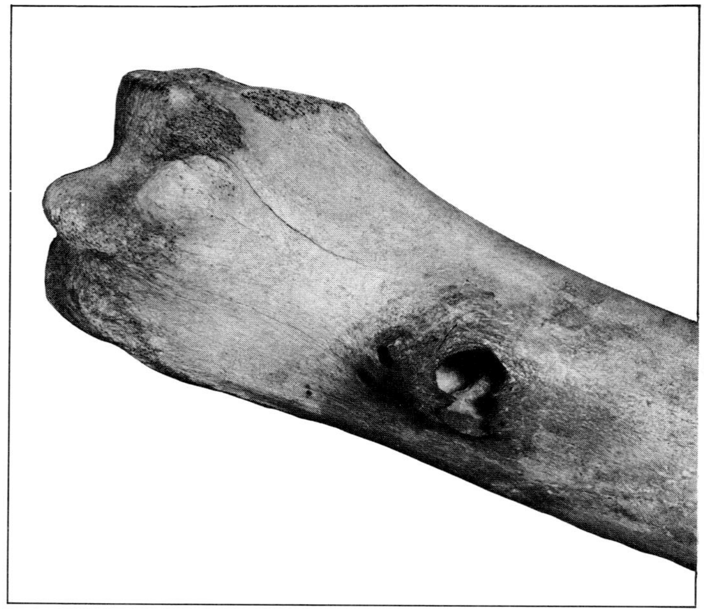

B A diseased bone from about two million years ago

One of the problems about studying prehistoric times is that we have no written evidence like **A**, so we have to make careful guesses from remains like **B**. But there are also problems with written evidence like **A**. The handwriting may be difficult to read, the writer may be biased (one sided), lie or make mistakes.

The way people live often affects the way medicine progresses. During wars, surgeons have often had to work out new ways of treating soldiers' wounds. Many of these new methods of operating have changed the ways in which surgeons worked after the war (see chapter 15). War has therefore brought about changes and improvements in medicine.

The ancient Egyptians believed that the human body would be needed after death. Priests would not allow surgeons to cut up or dissect bodies. Do you think this helped or slowed down doctors in learning about how the body worked?

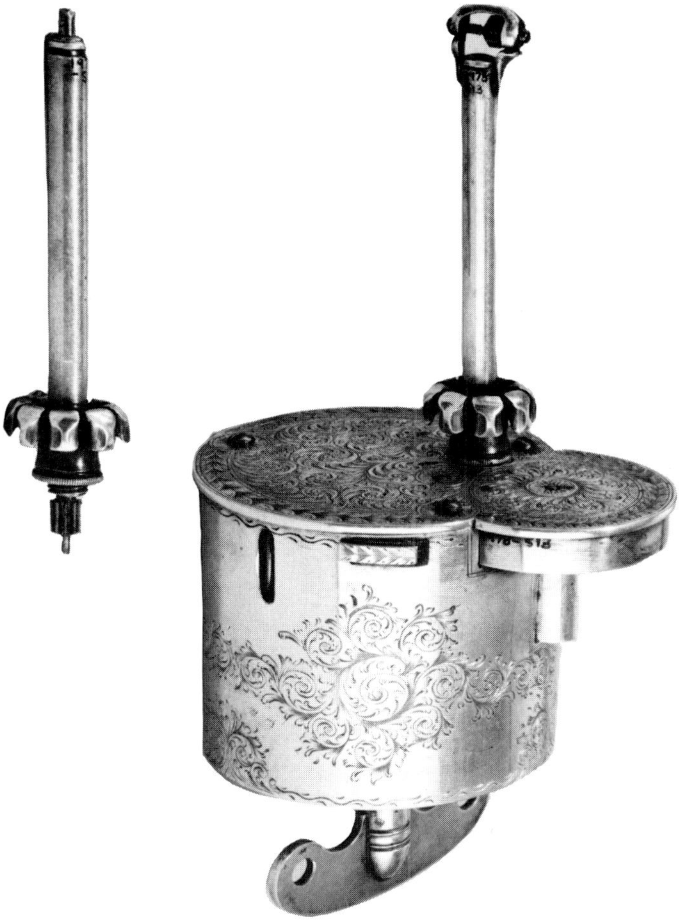

C Clockwork dental drill, 1870

D Model of the chemical workshop at the medical school in Alexandria

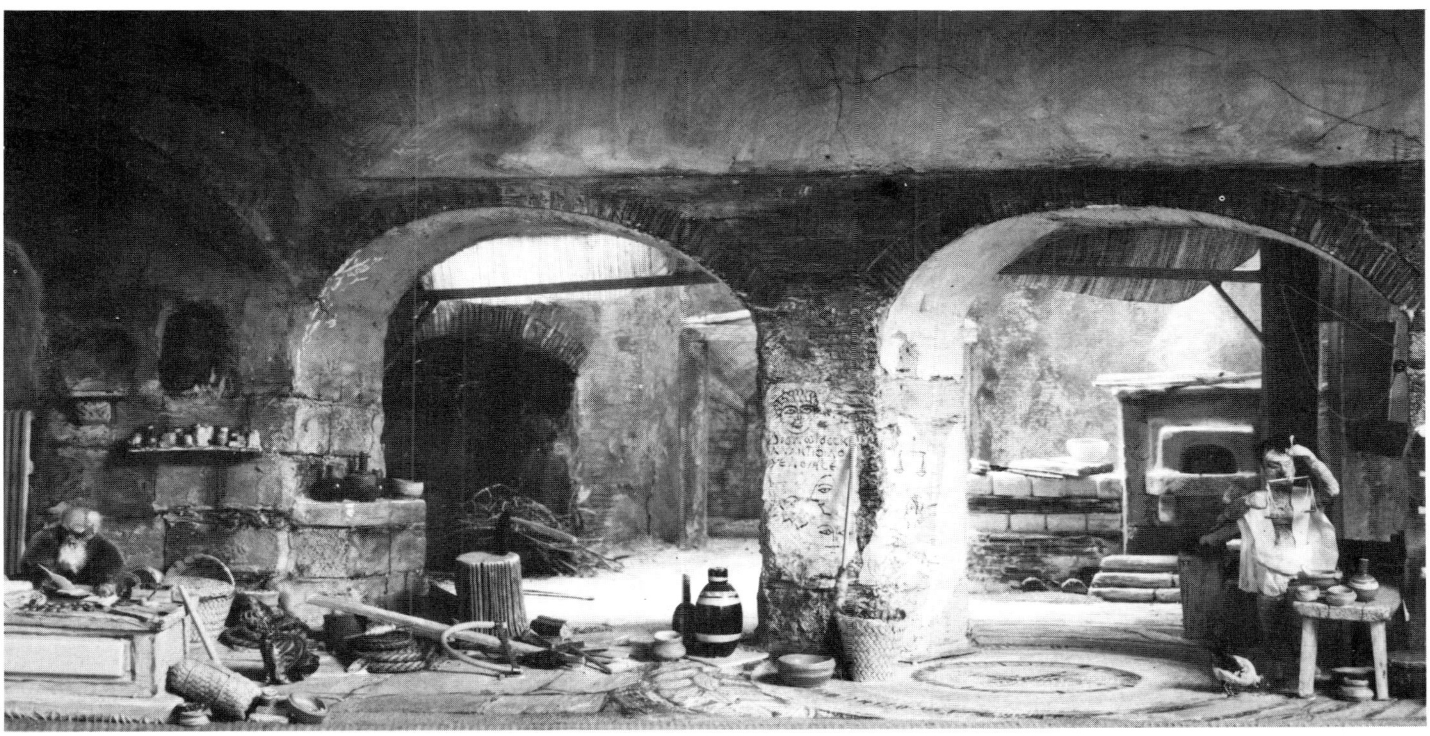

??????????????????

1 Look at sources **A** – **D**. Draw a chart like the one below and fill in the gaps:

	A	B	C	D
How was it written/made?				
Who wrote/made it?				
Is it a primary or secondary source?				
What value has the source for the historian?				
Can you trust what the source tells you?				

2 Give a primary and a secondary piece of evidence to go with each of these periods of time: Prehistoric times, Roman times, Middle Ages, World War Two, Today (clue – books, pictures, tools, etc.).

3 **D** is a secondary source. Explain what kind of sources the Science Museum might have consulted and used to produce it.

4 What kinds of evidence would you look at if you were trying to describe medicine in one of the periods listed in question 2?

1 Early Man and Medicine

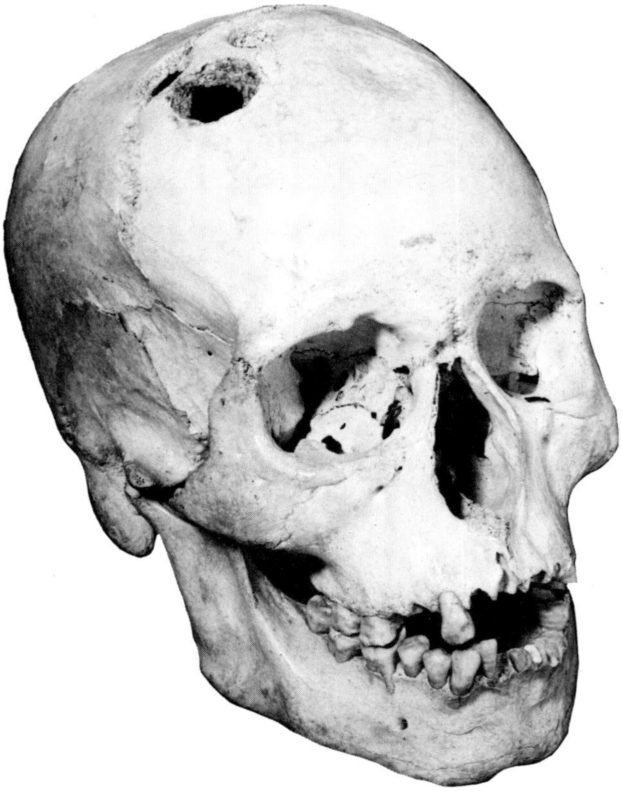

A Many such skulls have been found throughout Europe and the Middle East and archaeologists believe that the holes could not have been caused by accidents or fights. Skin had begun to form over many of the holes which showed that the people lived for some time after the holes had been made. These operations are called trepanning or trephining.

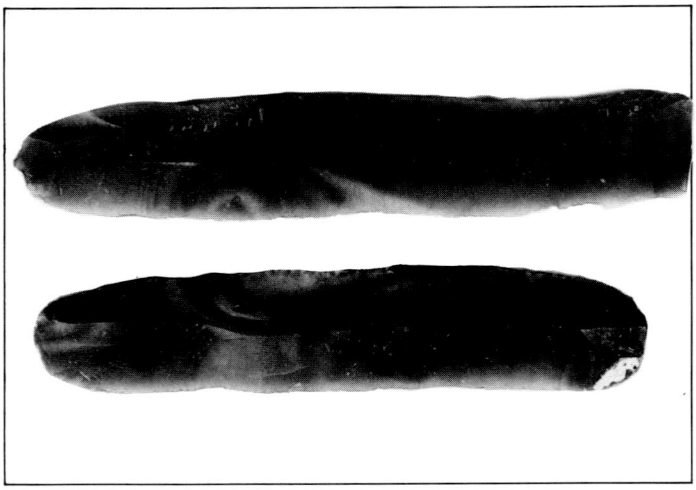

B Flint scrapers probably used to make the holes in trepanning

If you are ill and go to the doctor, how does he find out what is wrong with you? If you and the doctor wanted to find out about the illnesses of people who lived in prehistoric times (before man found out how to write), how would you go about it? You would have to look at the remains early man has left behind, such as **A–C.**

Scientists can tell us from clues found by archaeologists that very few prehistoric people lived beyond the age of thirty. They have worked this out from studying the bones and skulls of early man. Can you think how? We do not know why early man carried out operations like **A** (trepanning or trephining) or what people believed about medicine because we do not have enough evidence. One way to find out more is to look at present day primitive societies. If we know why primitive people, like the Aborigines, behave in the way they do we can perhaps understand some of the evidence that prehistoric people left behind. Prehistoric people's lives were like those of primitive tribes today. Most primitive tribes believe in magic or spirits. This belief affects how they practise medicine.

The Aborigines think that the rocks, seas and rivers are spirits that control the world. If a man is ill, the Aborigines say that an evil spirit may have entered his body, or that his own spirit has been drawn out of his body by an enemy. The Plains Indians of North America tell us that the earth is their Great Spirit. If they are ill, it means that the Great Spirit is angry with them. The San Blas islanders of the West Indies have medicine men. A 1969 school textbook on religion says:

The medicine man of the San Blas islanders in the West Indies possessed strange powers of healing. He made his medicines from herbs, berries and roots. However, instead of giving the medicine to the patient, he would take a small wooden doll and file pieces off the part of the body where the patient felt greatest pain. The wooden filings were mixed in water and the mixture was drunk by the patient. As with most primitive tribes the medicine men muttered a chant suitable for that particular illness. These San Blas islanders also believed that their medicine men had miraculous powers over storms and that they could walk on the clouds and even descend into the underworld.

How many of you wear a lucky charm or St Christopher? Today some primitive people wear lucky charms like **D** to keep away evil spirits. Archaeologists have found bones and teeth with holes drilled through them that people in prehistoric times wore.

Prehistoric man may also have used chants to make people better. A chant from ancient Sumeria goes:

Seven are they: seven are they:
In the ocean deep, seven are they:
Living in heaven, seven are they;
Bred in the depths of the ocean.
Neither man nor woman are they,
But are as the blast of the roving wind,
No wife have they, nor son can they beget,
They know neither mercy nor pity,
They listen not to prayer or pleading,
They are as wild horses from the hills.

We can also guess that early man may have used plants, roots and berries as medicine. Today one of our drugs for malaria, quinine, is based on its first use by ancient tribes in Peru.

Until man worked out that there were natural rather than supernatural causes of illness, progress was very slow in medicine and surgery. Until people found out that they could control and cure illness and disease they went on using the old methods such as spells, incantations, trepanning and the wearing of lucky charms and bracelets.

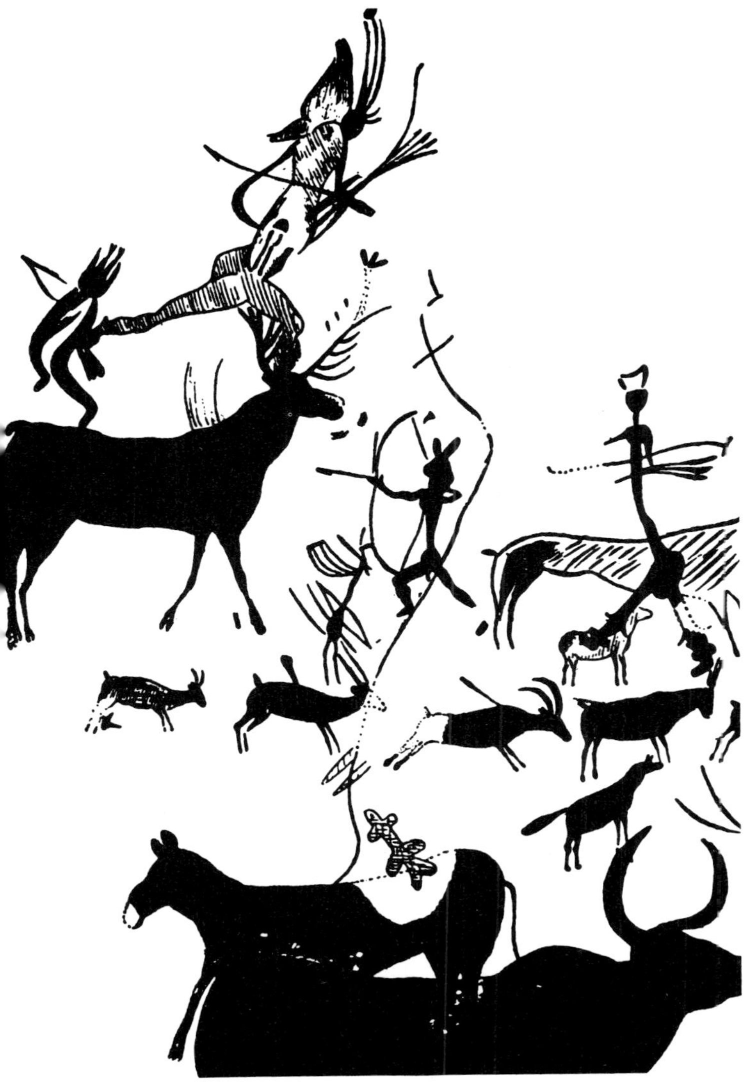

C Cave painting showing animals being hunted

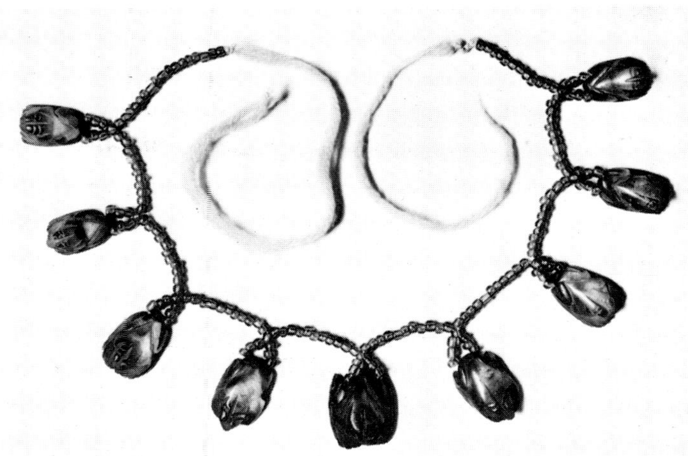

D Lucky charm worn by primitive tribes today

??????????????????

1 In pairs or groups discuss each of the sources **A–D.** For each produce *one* idea of what it suggests to you about early disease and medicine.

2 Match one of the sources **A, B** or **C** with one of the ideas below about early medicine:
Idea 1: flint knives and scrapers could have been used to make holes in the skulls of early man.
Idea 2: if prehistoric man had a headache he might believe that an evil spirit had entered his head, and that the best way to let out the evil spirit was to cut a hole in the skull.
Idea 3: early man painted pictures of animals on the walls of caves as an early form of magic to help him capture the animal when he hunted it.

3 If you had an accident today and had to go to hospital, a team of nurses and doctors would treat you. Imagine that you fell and broke your leg in prehistoric times. Describe what would happen to you until you were cured. Say what thoughts and fears you would have, and what methods might be used to treat you. Remember you might well have violent headaches during your illness, and something would have to be done about them.

4 Which of **A–D** are primary and which secondary sources? How much trust can you put in the sources **A–D** as *evidence* about how early man practised medicine?

2 Egyptian Medicine 3000-400 BC

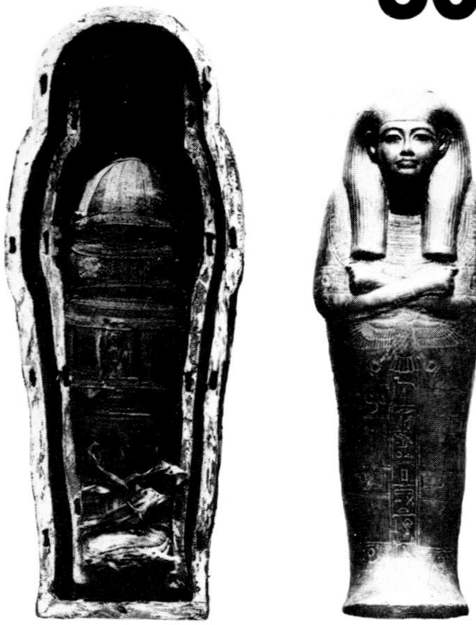

A Bodies were wrapped in bandages spread with a special powder to preserve them. The Egyptians believed people would need their bodies again in an after-life.

Just over a hundred years ago, archaeologists found a tomb in Egypt where the wife of a pharaoh (one of the kings of ancient Egypt) had been buried since about 2500 BC. The body was intact and had not rotted away because the Egyptians had turned it into a mummy before it was buried (see **A**). The archaeologists found paintings like **B** on the walls of the tomb and a medicine chest next to the body. In the chest were six jars that had the dried remains of drugs inside them, plus some spoons and dried roots. These things were all packed in a basket ready to be used in case of illness. Also in the chest the archaeologists found some scrolls of papyrus, an early kind of paper. The scrolls tell us about two famous doctors, Sekhetenach, who healed the king's damaged nostrils, and Imhotep (see **C**).

Other scrolls tell us about the cures Egyptian doctors used. One begins with a spell like **D** that was said when

B Tomb painting showing Anubis, god of death, preparing a mummy.

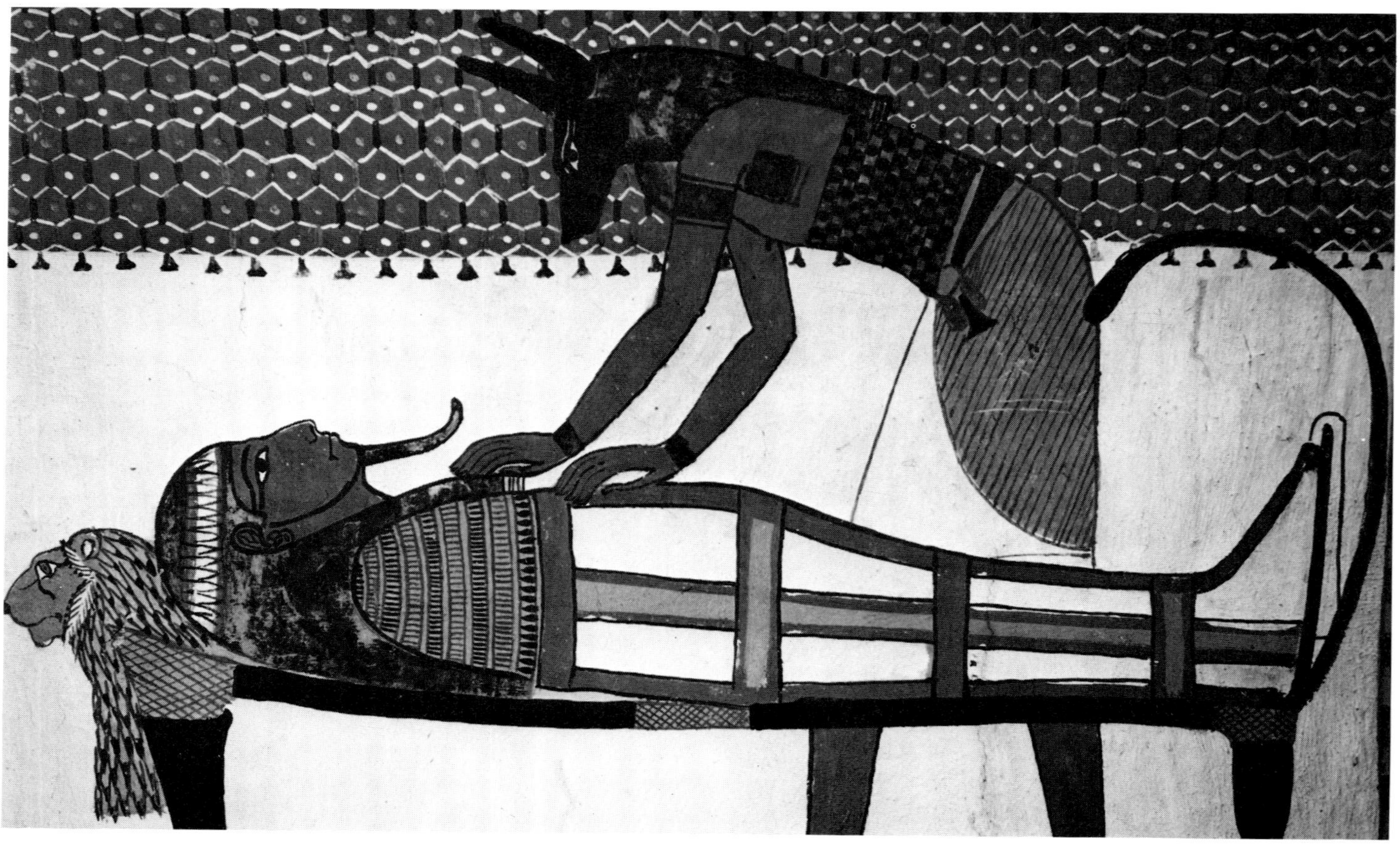

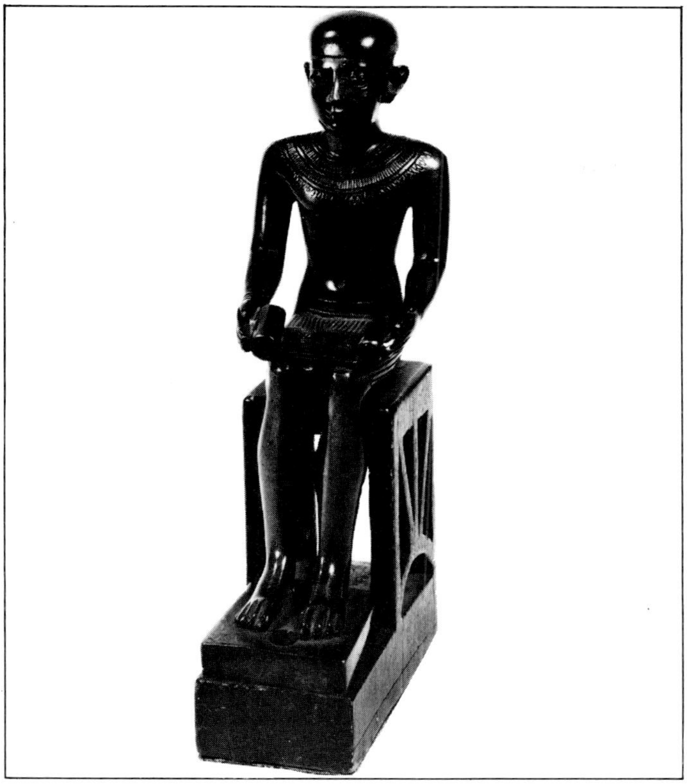

C Imhotep became a famous doctor of the Pharaohs and hundreds of years after his death people worshipped him as god of healing.

drinking a cure for an illness in the stomach:

‘ *Come. You who drive out evil things from my stomach and my limbs. He who drinks this shall be cured just as the gods above were cured.* ’ **(D)**

The papyrus scrolls describe about 700 cures for many illnesses. How would you like to try this cure? It is meant to help cure blindness.

‘ *A pig's eye, stibium, red ochre and a little honey are finely ground and mixed together and poured into the patient's ear.* ’ **(E)**

Despite such ideas, Egyptian doctors did have a clear view of how the human body worked. The papyrus tells us what we now know about the heart:

‘ *There are vessels from it to every limb. When any doctor, any surgeon or any exorcist* (a person who drives out evil spirits) *applies the hands or the fingers to the head, to the hands, to the parts of the stomach, then he also examines the heart because all the patient's limbs contain its vessels.* ’ **(F)**

By the fifth century BC there were many doctors in Egypt. Herodotus, the Greek historian, wrote:

‘ *Each doctor is a doctor of one disease and no more, and the whole country is full of physicians, for some say they know about eyes, others teeth, others the head, others illnesses of the stomach, others more rare diseases or ailments.* ’ **(G)**

Herodotus also wrote that the Egyptians knew about hygiene (keeping clean):

‘ *They drink from cups of bronze which they clean daily. They take extra care always to wear newly washed linen clothes. . .twice a day and every night the priests wash in cold water.* ’ **(H)**

Egyptians used to wash themselves often, using soda and scented oils.

Here are four reasons why the Egyptians may have made so much progress in medicine:

1 They believed that the body would be needed in a second life. So they took out some of the organs from a dead body and preserved them in jars. For example, the brain was taken out through the nostrils.
2 They had time to think about medicine because they lived in one place within a community.
3 They developed a new way of writing and were able to write down their ideas and findings on papyrus scrolls.
4 Their ships sailed to Southern Europe and Northern Africa where they could get drugs that the doctors needed, and learn about other people's medical ideas.

??????????????????

1 What do **E, F, G** and **H** tell us about Egyptian medicine? Work this out by yourself or talk about it in pairs.

2 Do sources **D, E** and **F** suggest that medicine in ancient Egypt was:
a scientific and sensible or
b based on superstitious beliefs?
What other information in the chapter backs up your answer?

3 Use all the information in the chapter to describe what a visit to a typical Egyptian doctor might have been like. Include the following words and phrases: I was blind. . .the physician was a specialist. . .he chanted a spell. . .he used the following remedy. . .the result was. . .

4 Which of the four reasons at the end of the chapter were the most important in improving Egyptian medicine? Put them in order of importance and give reasons for your choice.

3 Ancient Greece 800-300 BC

Do you believe in UFOs (Unidentified Flying Objects) or ghosts? Many people do. Or maybe you have heard of some strange event that no one can explain. Even today people believe in the supernatural. A supernatural cause is one which does not give a true reason, as we know it, to explain why things happen. For example, if you said, an 'evil spirit' or 'the devil' made you ill, that would be a supernatural reason.

The ancient Greeks believed in supernatural causes for things. For instance, they thought that different gods caused thunderstorms and winds. The Greeks looked for supernatural reasons to explain diseases. Many Greeks visited the temple of Asclepios, their god of healing, when they wanted to be cured (see chapter 4). They thought magical cures like the one in source **B** might happen in this temple:

❛ *A man had his toe healed by a serpent. When sleep came upon him a snake issued from the temple and healed the toe with his tongue.* ❜ (**B**)

A Mount Olympus: the throne of the great god Zeus and the home of the gods

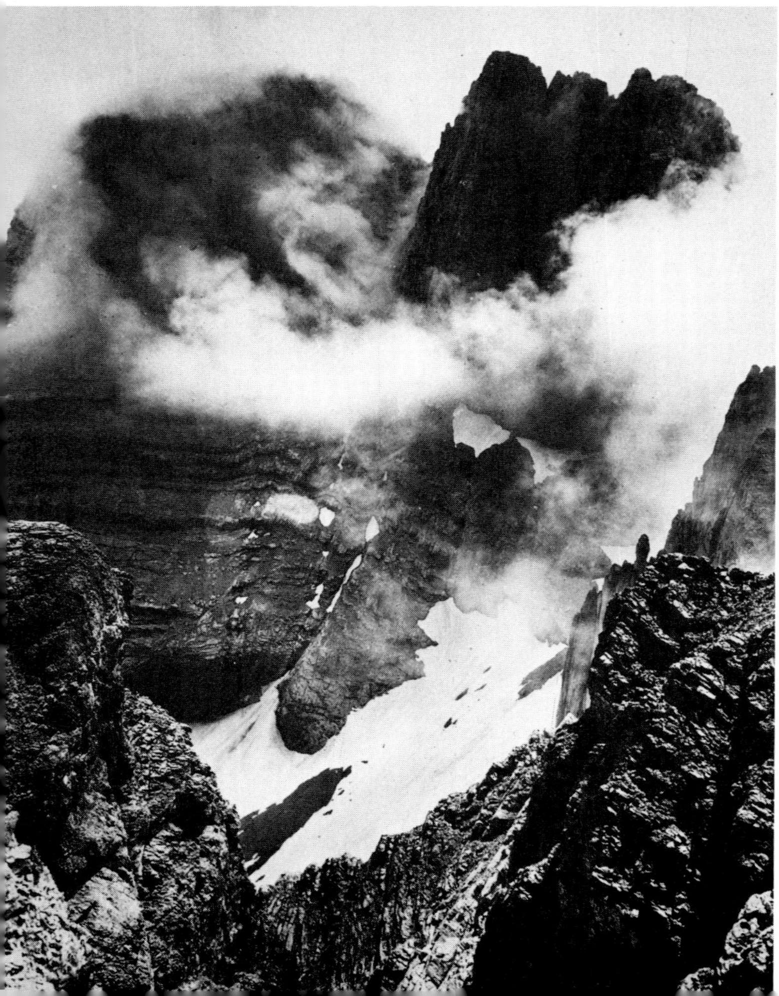

How often have you heard your mother tell you to wash behind your ears or clean your teeth? The same sort of advice was given by Greek doctors more than three thousand years ago. For instance Diocles of Christos, a Greek doctor, wrote in the fourth century BC:
Every day he should wash face and eyes and he should rub his teeth inside and out with his fingers.

Greek doctors believed that the best way to avoid falling ill was to keep fit by taking exercise. So, sports and games were a good way to stay healthy. This was one reason why the Greeks held so many athletics contests. The most famous was the Olympic Games, which were first held in about 776 BC (**C**).

Many Greeks lived in towns like Athens and Sparta. Each town had its school, and at Athens there was a

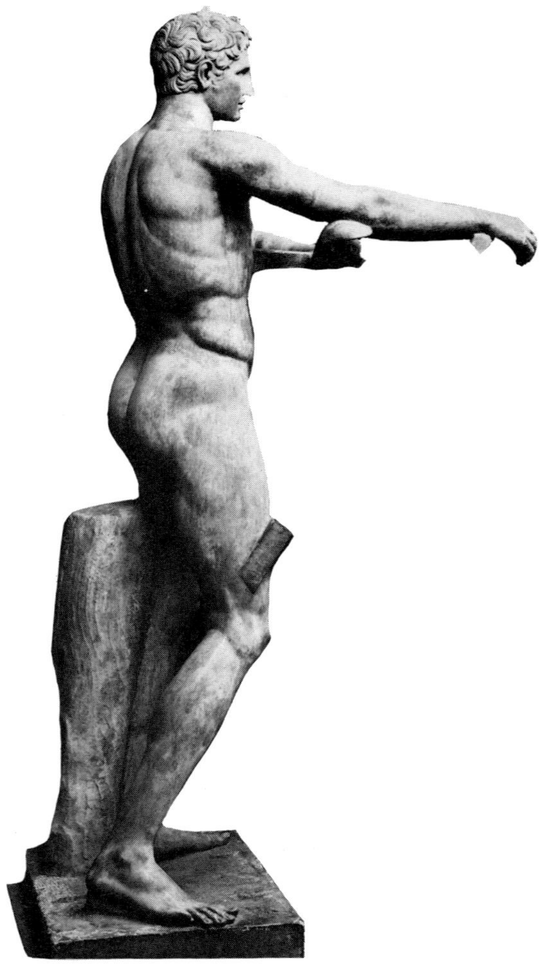

C An athlete from the ancient Olympic games. The competitors anointed themselves with oil as a protection against the hot sun because they always competed in the nude. This athlete is using a scraper called a strigil to remove the oil after an event.

famous school, the Academy. Greek teachers asked questions about all types of things. Between about 600 and 400 BC Greek thinkers in the towns began to try to find out *reasons* for why things happened in the world.. No longer were they happy to accept that the gods caused everything. Men like the Greek teachers and thinkers, Anaximander, Plato and Aristotle, started to look for natural reasons for what went on (**D**). For instance, Aristotle cut up or dissected animals and began to work out how their bodies functioned. At first the Greeks did not cut up human bodies because they thought the human body would be needed after death. But many doctors had looked closely at how human organs worked and at human bones when people were injured.

By about 300 BC Greek thinkers like Aristotle and Plato had convinced the Greeks that the human body was not needed after death, and so it could be dissected. Since the Greeks were also merchants and traded with Egypt, Greek doctors were able to learn a lot about Egyptian medicine from trade contacts.

D Busts of Plato and Aristotle

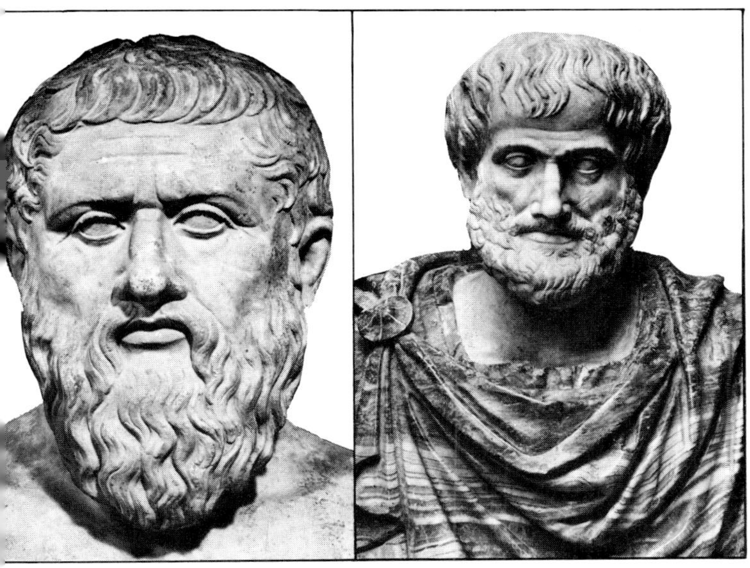

The School at Alexandria

Where the Greeks traded, settled and conquered they set up schools and universities. In 335 BC Alexander the Great conquered Egypt and built the Grecian city of Alexandria. There he founded a museum, library and famous university. Scholars, writers, philosophers and doctors all came to study at Alexandria. Here doctors could dissect dead bodies. One such surgeon, Herophilus, discovered that the brain, and not the heart, was in control of how the body moved. Another doctor, Erasistratus, found out that the heart pumped blood round the body. The famous Greek philosopher, Aristotle, taught many of the teachers at Alexandria university.

?????????????????

1 Put the following facts into their correct date order. Under each fact write one idea which that fact suggests to you about the history of medicine in Greece.

a 776 BC: Olympic Games first took place.
b 800 BC: Greek civilization began. Founding of towns and cities like Athens and Sparta.
c 600 BC onwards: Philosophers (thinkers) looked for natural explanations for events.
d 335 BC: Alexander the Great conquered Egypt and founded Alexandria.
e 350 BC: Greek doctors wrote about the need to keep fit.

2 *The Greeks made some contributions to the development of medicine but basically they still believed in the supernatural.*
What do you think? Write an essay about it, using the information below. There are five sentences in column A. You can use these as the opening sentences of five paragraphs in the essay. Decide in which order you will put the paragraphs and then look in column B for the block of information that goes with each sentence. The information in column B is in note form only. You should read the chapter again before writing the essay, and then write in full sentences.

Column A

1 The ideas of philosophers helped develop ideas in medicine.

2 The school of Alexandria also helped in the development of medicine.

3 Many Greek doctors realized the importance of keeping healthy.

4 The Greeks learnt so much about medicine and other things because. . .

5 Many Greeks, however, still believed in the supernatural.

Column B

prevent ill health. . .keep clean. . .exercise . . . Olympic games

farming. . .settled way of life. . .time to think about things. . .trade. . .ideas from other places

gods were the cause of thunder and lightening, etc. . . .Asclepios could cure in his temple. . .the human body was needed after death

thinking man began to ask why things happened instead of believing in gods . . . they decided the body was not needed after death

library. . .a place where writers and thinkers could meet. . .the discovery of the role of the brain took place there. . .human dissection was allowed

4 Asclepios

Have you heard of Lourdes in France (**A**)? Many people go there today because they have faith that the waters will cure them of their illnesses. Likewise, in ancient Greek times, people visited temples called Asclepaeia, where they worshipped the god Asclepios. Asclepios had been a Greek doctor. A legend tells that, because Asclepios was so good at healing the sick, the chief god, Zeus, became jealous and killed him with a thunderbolt. Over the centuries the Greeks began to worship Asclepios as the god of healing. At Epidaurus in Greece the people built a massive temple, called the Asclepaeia. The sick went there for Asclepios the god to cure them. Soon other Asclepaeia were built.

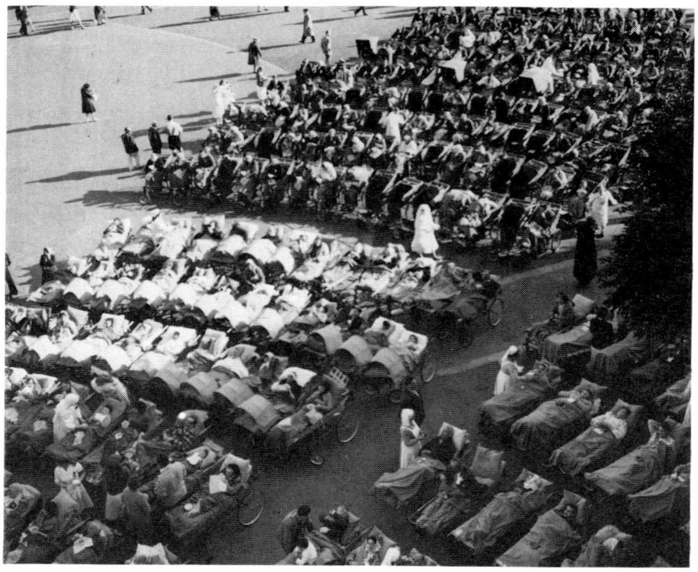

A Lourdes in France

The Greeks always built their Asclepaeia in healthy places near streams and in the countryside. Priests looked after the patients, whom they bathed and put on a diet. When the priests thought the time was right, they took the patient to a special room in the temple, the abaton. Once in the abaton, the patient was given drugs like poppy seeds or hemlock and went into a trance or half sleep. The priests dressed in white robes, and one of them would appear as Asclepios himself. The Greeks believed that serpents had special healing powers and tame serpents were used in the ceremony.

Some people seem to have been cured at the Asclepaeia. Archaeologists have found carvings and writings on the walls of the abaton which they think were placed there by people who had been cured (**B**). At first patients left gifts in the temple for the god Asclepios, but later many of the priests began to demand money.

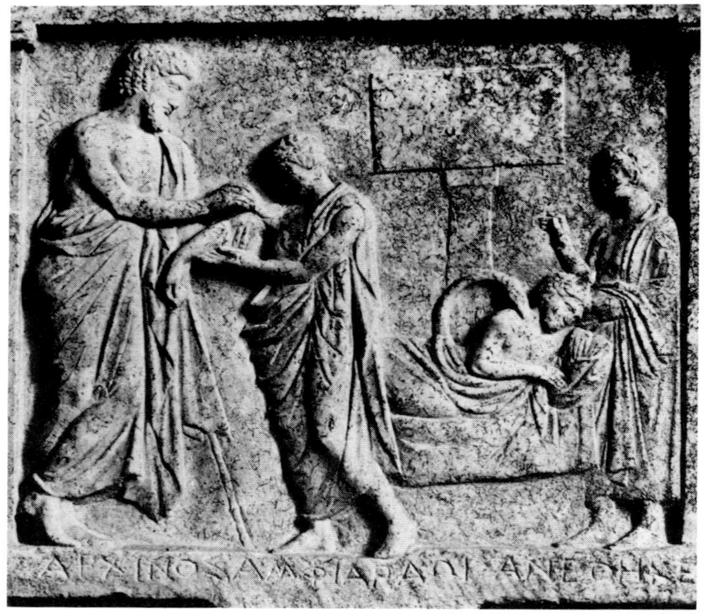

B A stone carving from an Asclepaeia shows the healing God (left) appearing to the dreamer. A serpent, supervised by a priest, climbs into the patient's bed and licks his wounds.

The worship of Asclepios was very widespread. As late as 293 BC the Romans began to worship Asclepios. They built an Asclepaeian temple on an island in the middle of the river Tiber. A legend tells us that a serpent had swum all the way from the temple at Epidaurus to the Tiber near Rome and cured someone of the plague.

???????????????????

1 a What is the link between **B** and Asclepios?

b What does the fact that the theatre at Epidaurus could seat 20,000 people suggest about the Asclepaeia there?

c Why do you think carved messages were put in the abaton for patients to read?

2 Imagine you are a Greek who visits the temple of Asclepios. Describe what happens to you. Include the following ideas:

Your illness. . .you decide to go to the Asclepaeia. . . your hopes. . .what happens when you arrive. . . your cure. . .you make up an inscription to place on the abaton wall.

5 Hippocrates

When we go to the doctor today, we take it for granted that he will listen to us, examine us, suggest things we can do or take to get better, make a note of our illness and ask to see us again to check that we are cured. We would also expect our doctor not to tell anyone else about our illness. Much of the way in which doctors today treat patients comes from the teachings of a Greek doctor called Hippocrates. He taught medicine at a small school on the island of Kos near Greece during the fourth century BC. He probably wrote the Hippocratic Oath which until recently all doctors had to swear to keep. Today, doctors take a very similar oath:

❛ *I will use treatment to help the sick according to my ability but never with a view to injury or wrongdoing . . . Whatever I see or hear professionally or in my private life, which ought not to be divulged, I will keep secret and tell no one.* ❜ **(A)**

Hippocrates lived at a time when the Greeks believed that the gods were the cause of illness and that only the gods or their priests could cure them. Hippocrates said:

❛ *Sickness is not sent by the gods or taken away by them. It has a physical basis. If we can find the cause we can cure the disease.* ❜ **(B)**

Our knowledge about Hippocrates comes from a series of books his students gathered together called the *Hippocratic Collection*. From these books we can see that Hippocrates turned medicine into a science. He taught that disease was a predictable process and that in order to cure a patient doctors must do four things:

1 *Diagnose*: look at a patient's symptoms to see what is affecting him. **(C)**

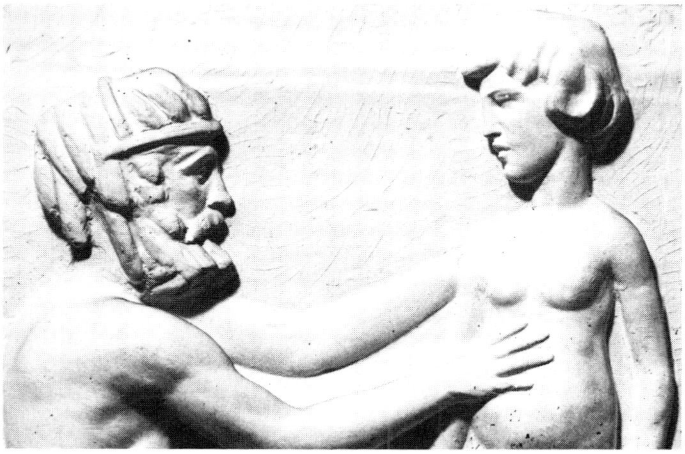

C This ancient Greek tablet shows a physician examining a patient.

2 *Make a prognosis*: make an informed guess about what is likely to happen if the illness comes on in the same way as illnesses like it.
3 *Observe*: look at and record the course of the illness.
4 *Treat*: if necessary give some treatment that will cure the illness.

This process is known as clinical observation. The methods are very similar to those that doctors use today (nearly 2000 years after Hippocrates). This is why Hippocrates is often called 'The Father of Modern Medicine'.

Hippocrates believed that the body was made up of four humours or liquids and that the seasons of the year affected the humours. If the humours become unbalanced, then the patient would become ill **(D)**.

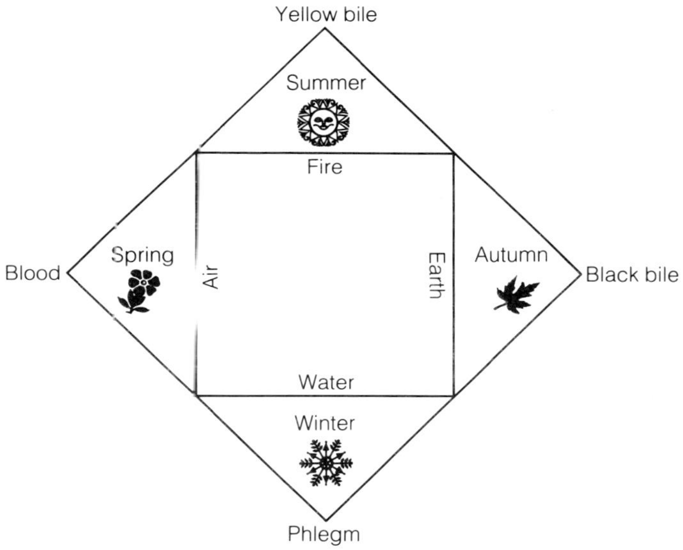

D The four humours of the body

??????????????????

1 How might Hippocrates have treated a patient who suffered from influenza? Make notes on each of the following: his diagnosis, prognosis, observation, treatment.

2 How might a follower of Asclepios have treated the same patient?

3 Use **D** to diagnose what might be wrong with patients who were:
a spitting blood; **b** producing bile.

6 Babylon, India and China

A

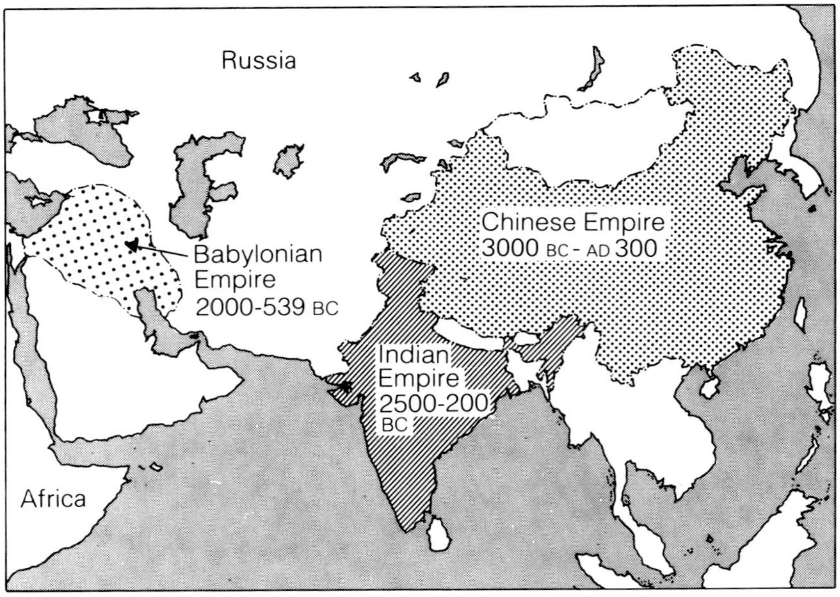

Babylon

Ancient civilizations other than Egypt's also had ideas about medicine. **B** shows a clay model of a sheep's liver which Babylonian doctors used for diagnosing illness. The Babylonians had a separate class of surgeons, known as Asu. In 1930 BC a Babylonian king, Hammurabi, wrote a code of laws. Here are some of the laws that apply to Asu or surgeons:

❛ *If a surgeon operates on a nobleman for a severe wound and saves the man's life . . . he shall receive a fee of ten shekels of silver. If the patient is a slave his master shall pay ten shekels of silver. However, if the doctor shall kill the patient or destroy the sight of an eye, his hand shall be cut off.* ❜ **(C)**

B Babylonian priest physicians made clay models of sheep's livers like **B.** Patients blew up the nose of a sheep. The sheep was then slaughtered and the physicians looked at the liver to diagnose the illness. Priest physicians would also consult the stars.

B

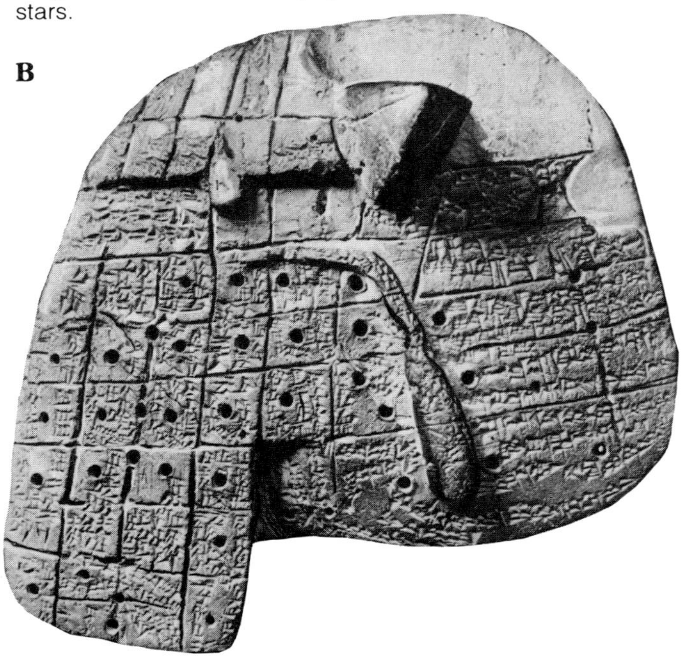

The Babylonians had many superstitious ideas. Surgeons could not operate on the seventh, fourteenth, twenty-first or twenty-eighth days of the month or in the seventh month of the year. Surgeons often wore frightful masks to scare away the demons of disease. But, one court doctor or physician, Arad-Nana, seems to have worked out something important about the spread of disease. He wrote to his master: *Beware flies and shun lice in the interests of good health.*

Archaeologists have found that Babylonian cities had drains and sewers. What does this suggest about the Babylonians and public health?

India

Between 2500 and 200 BC a rich civilization grew up in the valley of the Indus. The Indus civilization was based on cities. The city dwellers knew a great deal about the spread of disease. Archaeologists have found out that priest doctors lived in the cities and that they used spells, herbs and spices to get rid of disease.

Indian surgeons were skilled. They could repair a patient's nose by using a flap of skin taken from the forehead. Susruta, an Indian doctor who lived in AD 400 listed over 1000 surgical tools or instruments in use at that time. **D** is a clue about surgeon's work in ancient India. The thigh bones show marks of surgery.

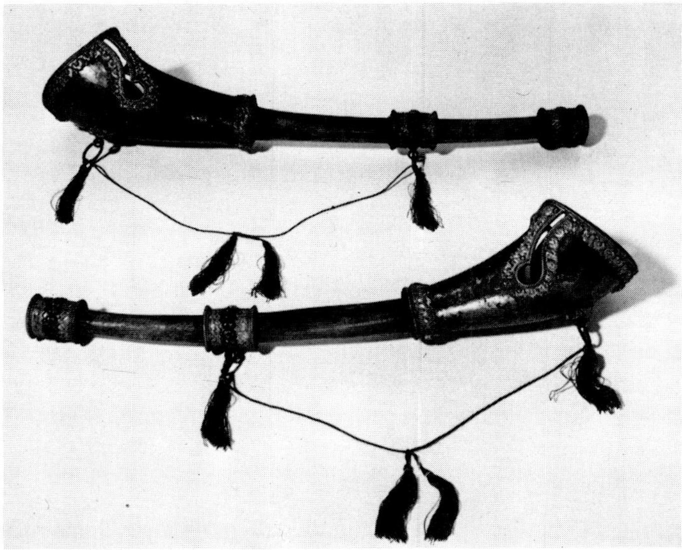

D A pair of Buddhist ritual trumpets: human thigh bones with silver and gilt mounts

F An ancient Chinese drawing showing acupuncture points

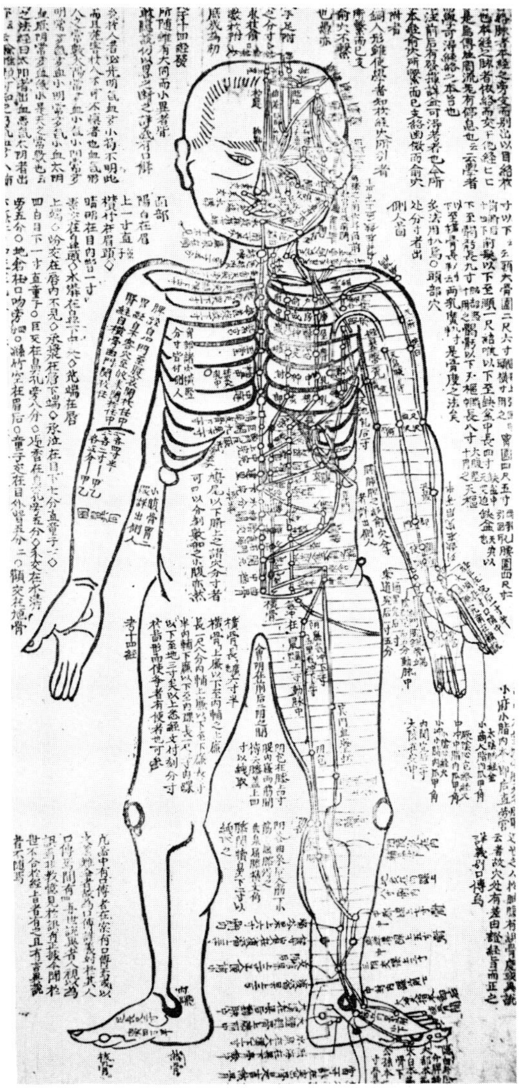

China

The ancient Chinese made many discoveries about medicine. These discoveries were made in China long before they were made in Europe. But China was so remote and cut off from the rest of the World that the discoveries did not become known outside China for a very long time. Emperor Shen Nung (about 3000 BC) listed over 100 drugs in a book. Many of these drugs are still in use today.

A book called *The Chinese Canon of Medicine* was written in about 2000 BC. This was long before the Egyptians developed a way of writing (see chapter 2). It tells how to take the pulse and explains how:

❛ *All the blood of the body is under the control of the heart and flows in a circle and never stops.* ❜ (**E**)

In Europe, William Harvey, an Englishman, did not discover that blood circulated round the body until 1628.

Hua Tu (AD 115–205) was a Chinese surgeon who used anaesthetics thousands of years before James Simpson discovered a suitable anaesthetic in Europe (see chapter 1). Chang Chung-Ching (AD 195) is known as the Chinese Hippocrates because he insisted that his students observe a patient's illness and study and record the symptoms of his disease for future use.

Acupuncture was developed by the Chinese and is still used today. Very fine needles are put into certain parts of the body in order to relieve pain and diseases, **F**.

??????????????????

1 Look at map **A** and then complete a time line like the one below by putting on the ancient civilizations of Babylon, China and India.

EGYPTIANS — GREEKS — ROMANS

3000 BC | **2000 BC** | **1000 BC** | **400 BC** | **0** | **400 AD** | **1000 AD**

2 Write a sentence or two about the importance of each of the following to the history of medicine: Hammurabi, Arad-Nana, Susruta, Shen Nung, Hua Tu, Chang Chung-Ching.

3 What does each clue **B–F** tell us about medicine in the ancient civilizations?

4 List two superstitious ideas about medicine shown in this chapter and two more sensible or scientific ideas.

5 Do you think **C** was a fair or unfair law? Would it have worked?

7 The Romans and Public Health 700 BC-AD 400

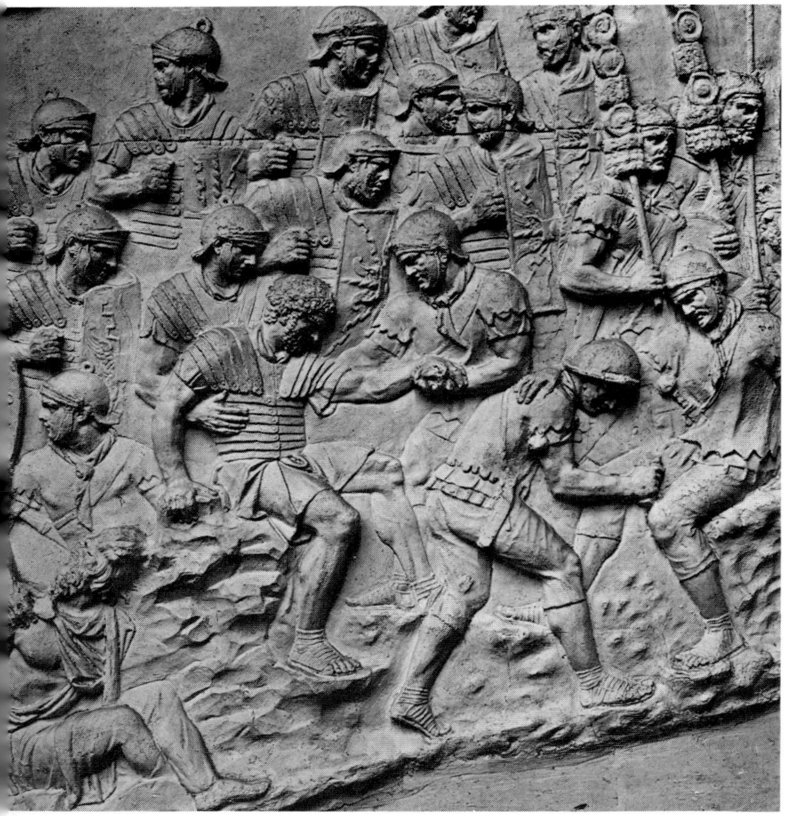

A A section from Trajan's Column shows soldiers treating the wounded.

What does evidence like **A** tell us about Roman doctors? By about 100 BC the Romans had conquered most of western Europe and North Africa. One reason why they had been able to do this was because they had a strong healthy army. We know that great care was taken to keep the soldiers fit because many Roman military hospitals have been found as far apart as Germany, Switzerland, Britain and North Africa. These hospitals were particularly healthy because they had drainage systems to take away the sewage. What does this suggest about the Romans' knowledge of cleanliness and health?

One Roman writer, Vegetius, wrote the following advice about how soldiers could keep healthy. The same advice would have been useful to any Roman citizen:

‘*Soldiers must not remain too long near unhealthy marshes . . . must not drink swampy water . . . daily exercise is better than physicians . . . If a group of soldiers is allowed to stay in one place too long in the summer . . . then they begin to suffer from the effects of polluted water and are made unhealthy by the smell of their own excrement. The air becomes unhealthy and they catch diseases.*’ (**B**)

The Romans seem to have taken great care about building towns that were healthy to live in. In the sixth century BC the *Cloaca Maxima* (main sewer) was built in

D The Claudian aqueduct near Rome

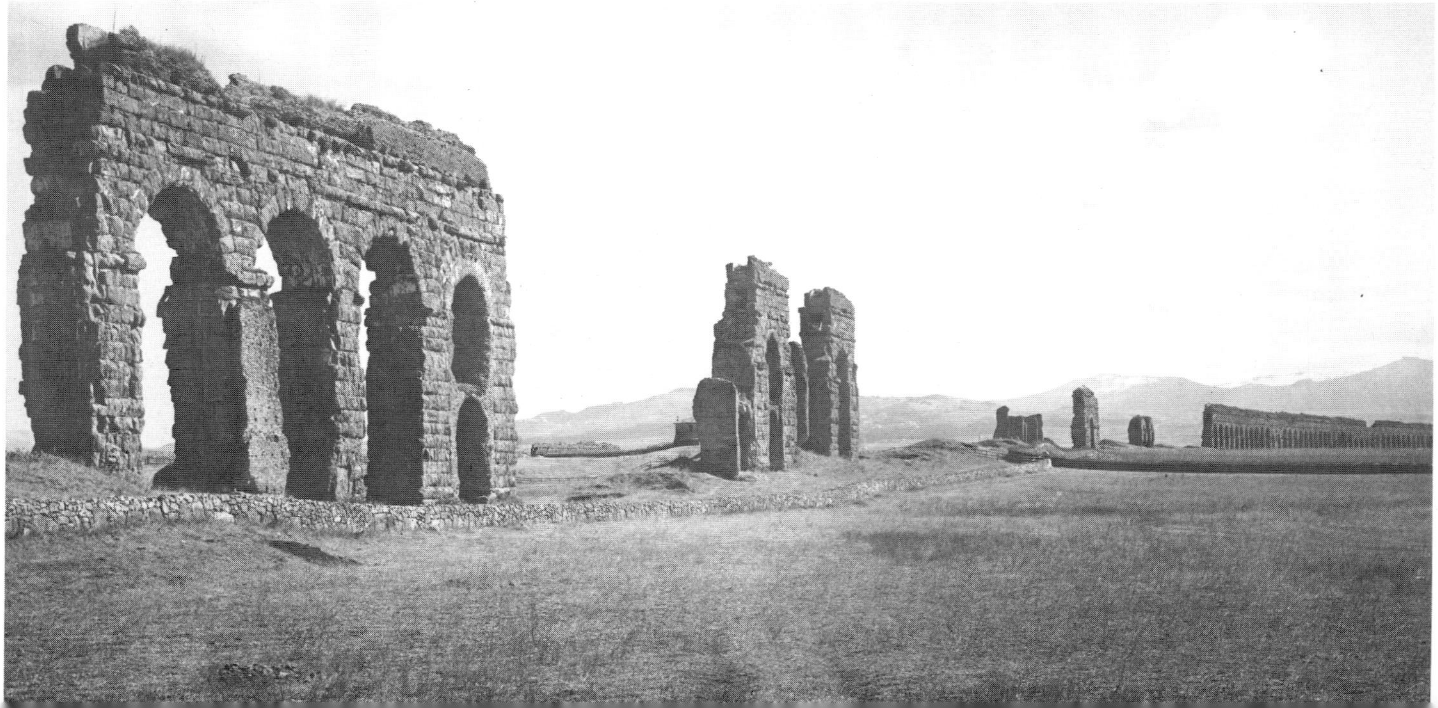

Rome to carry sewage out of the city. Julius Frontinius, a Roman writer, wrote the following in AD 42:

❛ *My job concerns not merely the convenience, but also the health of the city and so the task has always been handled by the most important men in the State.*

Now nine aqueducts bring water into the city. The aqueducts reach the city at different levels so that some deliver water to the high ground and some to the low ground. ❜ **(C)**

By the second century AD there were fourteen aqueducts like **D** bringing fresh water by pipes to the ground floor rooms of houses in Rome.

The Romans believed that keeping people and living conditions clean would keep people healthy. The rulers therefore tried to make the towns throughout the empire healthy places to live in.

Archaeologists looking at Roman towns as far apart as Bath in England and Pompeii in Italy have found remains like **E**, showing that Roman towns had a system of Public Health. The entrance fee to these baths was usually about the same as a penny today, so almost everyone could afford to go.

The Romans did not make the same progress in medicine as they had in public health. Doctors in Rome were not always thought of as being very good:

❛ *I'm ill, I sent for Semachus, he's here,*
A hundred students following in the rear;
All paw my chest with hands as cold as snow,
I had no fever but I have it now. ❜ **(F)**

Martial, a Roman poet AD 40-120

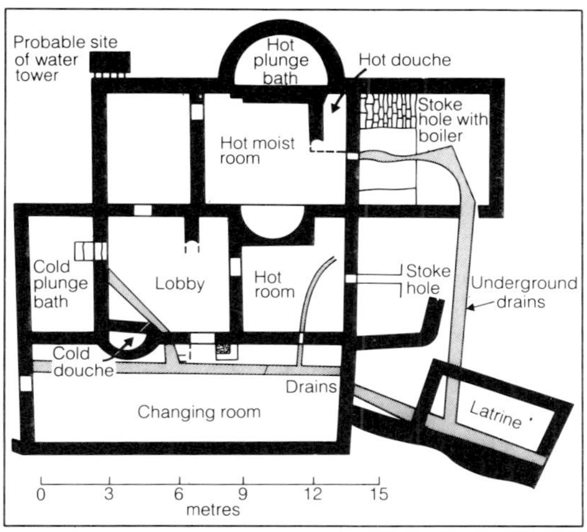

E Plan of the bath house at the Roman fortress at Vindolanda, Northumberland. The Roman writer Celsus suggested: 'If a man goes to the baths he should first stay wrapped up and sweat for a while in the tepidarium (warm room). Next he should go into the caldarium (hot room). After a further sweat . . ., he should have a shower first with hot, then tepid and then cold water.'

To become a doctor, all you had to do was put up a sign claiming you were a doctor. As a result, there were probably many very bad doctors. Many of them came from Greece and the Romans distrusted them. Can you think why?

Many people became doctors because doctors did not have to pay taxes. These doctors often offered totally different cures for the same illnesses and most of the cures did not work. The most common 'cure' was *theriac* which was made of about sixty different ingredients, the main one being snake's flesh.

All the changes made by the Romans improved the people's standard of health, which was a major achievement. However, the Romans did little to improve the treatment of disease. They virtually ignored the advances suggested by Hippocrates (see chapter 5) and still preferred to pray to gods like Asclepios rather than look for natural explanations for disease.

?????????????????

1 Copy and complete the chart below to show what **A-F** show us about medicine and public health in Roman times.

Source	Primary/ Secondary	Description	What it tells us about medicine and public health
A	Primary	Stone carving	Roman soldiers had surgeons to treat them and they also carried first aid kits.
B			

2 Look at **F**:
a What is the writer's opinion of doctors?
b What evidence is there in the chapter to support the writer?
c What evidence is there to contradict him?

3 Copy the diagram in **E.** Show with numbers and arrows the order that Celcus suggests for entering the rooms.
What evidence makes us think that even the poor people in Roman times could use the public baths?

4 Write a paragraph in answer to the question: 'In what ways did the Romans contribute to the development of medicine?'
Include the following words and phrases: the Roman Empire, the health of the army, military hospitals, siting of towns in healthy places, drainage and sewage, public baths, aqueducts.

8 Galen and Anatomy AD 130-200

Claudius Galen was born in Pergamon in Greece in AD 130. By the age of 21 he had studied in Smyrna and Alexandria (see chapter 3) and had written half a dozen books on medicine. He then travelled for nine years studying in the great medical centres of Corinth, Phoenicia, Palestine, Crete and Alexandria. When he returned to Pergamon he became chief doctor or medical officer at the amphitheatre where gladiators fought (**A**). He learnt much about the human body by having to treat the wounds of the gladiators. Human dissection was forbidden so this was one of the few ways in which Galen could learn about the body. (The study of the structure of the body is called anatomy.)

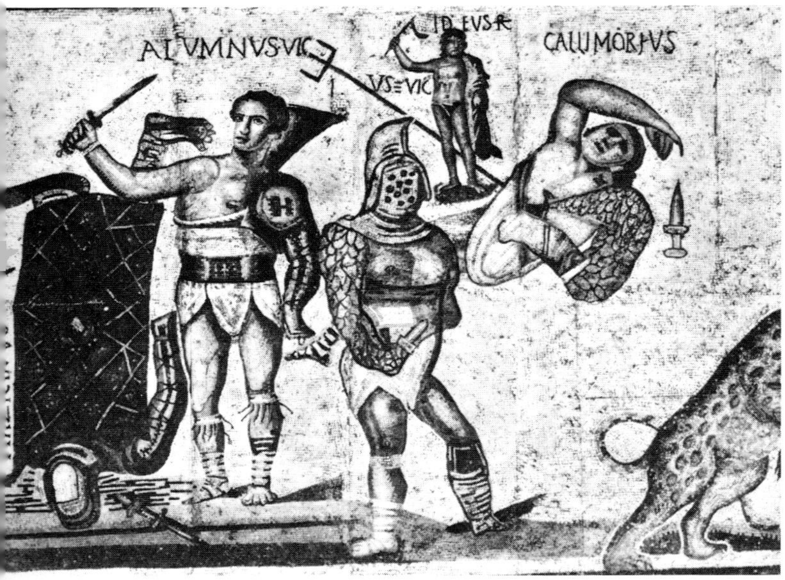

A A Roman mosaic showing gladiators fighting

There is some evidence that Galen once dissected the corpse of a drowned man, but he gained most of his knowledge by dissecting animals such as pigs, dogs and apes (see **B**). He assumed that humans were put together in the same way as apes, as this passage from his writings shows:

❛ *You can dissect an ape and learn each of the bones from it . . . For this you must choose apes that mostly resemble men . . . in these apes which also run and walk on two legs, you will also find the other parts as in man.* ❜ (**C**)

From* On Anatomical Procedures, *book 1, chapter 2

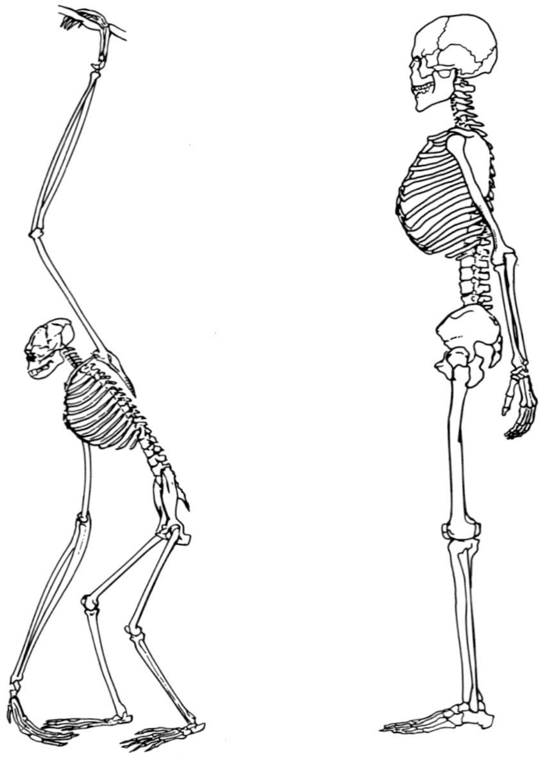

B Skeletons of gibbon and man

At the age of 32 he went to Rome and openly criticized the doctors there. Galen said they were ignorant, charged too much and gave the profession a bad name. He became physician to three emperors after he had cured the emperor Marcus Aurelius of a stomach ache. He developed bandaging methods that were used for centuries, worked out a theory about the movement of blood through the lungs and carried out experiments on the nervous system. People regarded Galen as an expert because he often made statements like this one:

❛ *Never yet have I gone astray whether in treatment or prognosis as have so many other physicians of great repute. If anyone wishes to gain fame . . . all that he needs is to accept what I have been able to establish.* ❜ (**D**)

For over a thousand years doctors and physicians thought Galen was right about medicine. He believed in only one God, so Christians and Arabs were happy with his teaching. Even as late as 1539, more than 1300 years after his death, the College of Physicians in London asked a doctor, John Geynes, to apologize when he suggested that some of Galen's work contained mistakes.

9 The Dark Ages AD 400-1100

During the fifth century the Roman Empire broke up because of attacks by tribes like those shown on map **A.** In Europe, for centuries after this, progress in medicine was halted. The tribes did not live in towns, so the Romans' knowledge of Public Health was not used. This was the start of the *Dark Ages*. Very little learning went on in Europe because most of the books were scattered or destroyed. This made it difficult for people to study subjects like medicine. Faith and belief in magic became popular again, as they had been before Roman times.

A

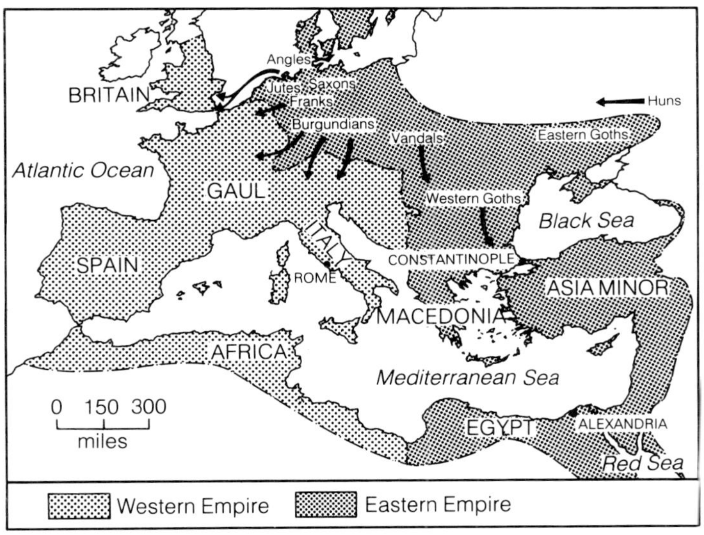

Here is a cure for epilepsy written during the Dark Ages:

❛ *Take a nail of a wrecked ship, make it into a bracelet and set therein the bone of a stag's heart taken from its belly whilst alive; put it on the left arm; you will be astonished at the result.* ❜ **(B)**

The church had a great influence on ideas. It taught that disease was a punishment from God and that the only way to be cured was to pray. Martyred saints became patron saints of parts of the body, depending on how they had been tortured. St Erasmus had his intestines torn out which made him the protector against intestinal trouble.

It was only in the monasteries that ideas about medicine and hygiene were kept alive. **C** is from a description of the monastery of Canterbury in about 1080. What does it tell us about the monks' standard of hygiene?

❛ *In the time before Christmas the monks are allowed to bath. Those who want to can shave and then take a change of clothes and go to the place where the baths are prepared. They then undress in the same order as they do in the dorter* (bedroom) *and go into the bathing place when they are told. They let down the curtain and sit in silence in the bath. If anyone wants anything, he must make a sign and a servant will bring it.* ❜ **(C)**

St Benedict, founder of the Benedictine monks, thought that the cure of the sick was one of the most important duties of a monk, and monasteries became the only hospitals in Europe during the Dark Ages. Some of the books on medicine by Greek and Roman writers were kept in the monasteries. Most of these books, such as Pliny's *Natural History,* were written in or translated into Latin. All monks throughout Europe read Latin and so they could learn much from these books. Most of the important Greek books on medicine were unfortunately lost to scholars in Europe at this time. Copies of these books, however, survived in the Arab Empire (see chapters 10 and 11).

??????????????????

1 Write a paragraph about all Galen's achievements. Include the following words: books, amphitheatre, dissections, bandages, blood, nervous system.

2 Look at **B** and **C** on p. 16. What did Galen assume about men and apes? What should Galen have learned from **B** about the human body?

3 What evidence is there that Galen studied Hippocrates (chapter 5)?

4 Rewrite this paragraph leaving out the phrases that you think are wrong:
The Dark ages was a period of time when it seemed that *not very much/great* change was taking place in medicine. People seemed to have *learnt/not to have learnt* much since the time of the Romans. The *Arab/Roman* Empire had *broken up/increased in size*. This meant that, whereas previously the Romans had been *able/unable* to spread their ideas about Public Health, now there was no strong empire to carry this out in Europe.

5 Say how each of the following had an effect on the development of medicine during the Dark Ages: **a** the breaking up of the Roman Empire; **b** the beliefs of the Christian Church; **c** the monasteries.

10 Centres of Medicine in the Dark Ages

During the Dark Ages in western Europe, learning lived on in the Arab schools and universities such as those of Cordoba (Spain) and Syracuse (Sicily). The Koran, the Muslim holy book, encouraged the study of medicine: 'O servant of God, use medicine because God hath not created a pain without a remedy for it.' So the Arabs set up schools of medicine as well as hospitals. This was partly due to the efforts of Nestorius, a Roman.

In AD 431 Nestorius, the Bishop of Rome, fled to Jundi-Shapur in Persia. He brought with him some scrolls of Greek writers such as Hippocrates. Many more scrolls were brought to Jundi-Shapur and translated into Arabic. Later, the library was moved to Baghdad, where a paper-making factory was set up in the eighth century.

The Arabs built at least thirty hospitals in places like Baghdad, Damascus and Cordoba. The most important was at Cairo, where there were separate wards for men and women and for the treatment of different diseases, such as eye complaints (**A**). Students studied there under famous physicians.

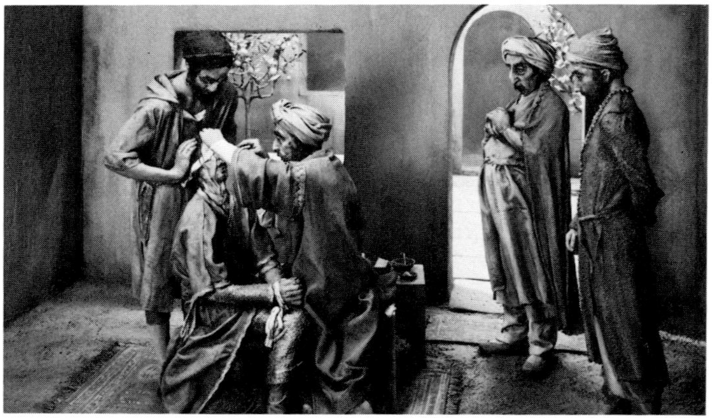

A Eye surgery in the eleventh century in Persia.

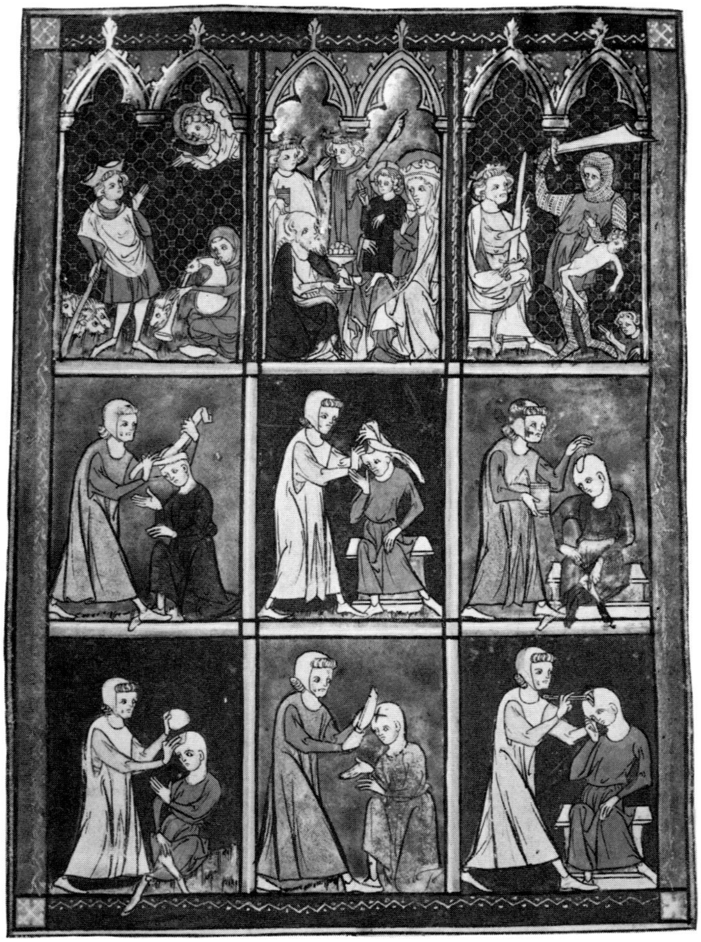

B From the *The Book of Surgery* by Master Roger of Salerno in the thirteenth century. It shows a physician treating different kinds of wounds and ailments.

In 1258 Baghdad was attacked and the Muslim Empire came to an end. By then, a famous medical school had grown up at Salerno, thirty miles south of Naples in Italy. Men and women of all races could study anatomy there, although only animals were dissected. Under Roger II of Sicily (1130-54), Salerno's medical school had a curriculum, qualifying examinations and degrees. The students began with a three-year course in logic, followed by two years of anatomy and surgery and a year of practice under an experienced doctor. Salerno was the first place to use the term 'Doctor of Medicine'. A famous book on surgery (**B**) was written at Salerno in the thirteenth century. The *Regimen Sanitatus Salemitatum* is another famous book from Salerno. It gave advice in rhyme on how to keep healthy:

‘ *Nor trivial count it after pompous fare,*
To rise from table and to take the air,
Great suppers will the stomach's peace impair;
Would'st lightly rest? – curtail thine evening fare. ’ (**C**)

The idea of medical schools spread from Salerno to the rest of Europe. Later, there were medical schools built at Boulogne, Montpellier and Naples, and at the universities of Paris, Padua, Oxford and Cambridge.

11 Rhazes, Albicasis, Avicenna and Arab Medicine

The Arab Empire spread across most of the Middle East and North Africa. The Arabs made advances in medicine at a time when the rest of Europe was in the Dark Ages. Three of the most famous Arab doctors were Rhazes, Albicasis and Avicenna.

Rhazes lived from about AD 860-932. He hung up fresh meat in various parts of the city of Baghdad, and built a hospital where the meat took longest to start to rot. At the Baghdad hospital Rhazes taught students to observe their patients' symptoms and he worked out the difference between smallpox and measles. He wrote over 150 books on medicine, one of which was an encyclopaedia that weighed 10 kilograms. Rhazes was such a famous teacher that people came from all over the Arab Empire to hear him lecture. In turn, he made trips to North Africa, Egypt and India to gather knowledge about illnesses and how to cure them. All the money that Rhazes earned he gave to the poor and he died a poor man.

Albicasis (936-1013) wrote books on both medicine and surgery, which included illustrations of many surgical instruments that were used at the time. He used the cautery to cure more than 50 diseases. This was an iron bar that was heated and used to seal wounds and stop infection. He revived surgery when it was an almost forgotten art. Albicasis was also a dentist and carried out operations to straighten ugly teeth.

Picture **A** shows Avicenna, 980-1037, another Persian doctor. Avicenna became a court doctor or physician at the age of 18. In his search for herbs and medicine he visited many cities. Then he became a teacher and doctor at the court of Cordoba in Spain. He wrote *The Canon of Medicine* which became the standard textbook on medicine for doctors for the next 400 years.

A Avicenna

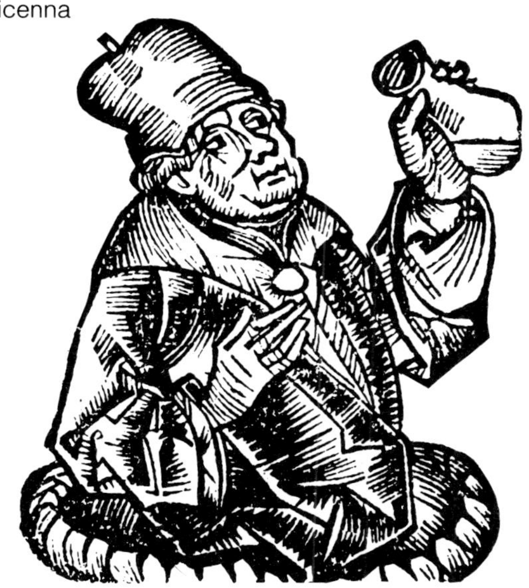

The Arabian drug store

How many different kinds of drugs and medicine are on sale at your local chemist? The Arabian Empire was where chemist's shops began. Doctors as well as ordinary people could buy herbs and medicinal plants collected from all over the empire, including alcohol, cassia, senna, manna, arsenic and many more. We make our pills taste nice by coating them in sugar; the Arabs did the same thing by using rosewater and perfumes. The chemist's shops also had on sale the first plasters and ointments to be used.

???????????????????

1 a Why was learning about medicine more likely to take place under the Muslim religion than under Christianity during the Dark Ages?

b How were the works of Greek writers preserved during the Dark Ages?

c How might the setting up of a paper factory help to spread ideas about medicine?

2 a Look at the evidence on p. 18. What does **A** tell us about the standard of hospitals and surgery in the Arab Empire in the eleventh century?

b Describe what the pictures in **B** are trying to show.

c Write, in your own words, the advice given in **C.** Do you think it is good advice? Say why.

3 Read carefully chapters 9, 10 and 11 and then answer this essay question.

Most major developments in medicine during the years 400-1100 took place in the Muslim Empire. Discuss these developments and the reasons for them.

Include the following in your answer; the effect of the Christian religion; the effect of the Muslim religion; centres of learning in Europe and the Arab Empire; the work of individuals such as Nestorius, Rhazes, Avicenna, Albicasis; the development of drugs.

12 The Doctor in the Middle Ages 1100-1500

In western Europe, in contrast to the Muslim Empire, the standard of doctors was very low during the Dark and Middle Ages.

❛ *I know that doctors besiege your bedside, and naturally this fills me with fear. Their opinions are always conflicting. As Pliny said, in order to make a name for themselves they gamble with our lives . . . They learn their art at our expense . . . O most Gentle Father, look upon their band as an army of enemies. Remember the warning epitaph which that unfortunate man has written on his tombstone: I died of too many physicians.* ❜ (**A**)

Petrarch (1304-74) an Italian poet, wrote **A** to a Pope who was ill. Petrarch's opinion of doctors could be based on evidence such as **B** (advice to doctors written by John of Ardennes):

❛ *First, he must put God first and always ask for his help. He should ask of a worthy man £40, with a robe and fee* (on top) *of 100 shillings . . . , of less men £40 ask he (but) without fees and take he not less than 100 shillings. For never in my life took I less than 100 shillings* (£200 in modern day money) *for the cure of a sickness.* ❜ (**B**)

Here are some 'cures' that typical doctors of the time might offer. All these 'cures' were used and most people accepted them as the best possible treatment.

For toothache: hang the beak of a magpie round your neck.
For a headache: put goat's cheese on the head.
For a fever: use a leech to suck blood from the arm.

What do these 'cures' suggest about doctors' knowledge of the teaching of men like Hippocrates? Do they show a scientific or a superstitious approach to medicine?

Surgery was also in a poor state. Students of surgery in the Middle Ages dissected pigs to learn about the workings of the human body. Some were able to practise on the bodies of soldiers or knights killed in battle. They usually pulled out the organs that would come out most easily. **C** is a redrawing of the earliest known picture of such a dissection. Above the body are the heart, lungs, kidneys and stomach and the man with the knife is holding the liver. But only army surgeons could get this much experience.

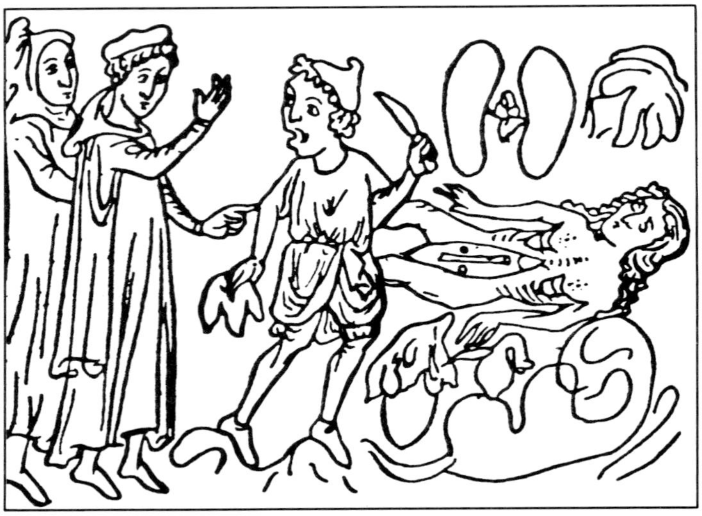

C A re-drawing of the earliest known picture of a dissection of a soldier killed in battle.

'Surgeons' tended to do the job part-time and treated only minor wounds. Their main job would have been as a barber or a butcher and the most popular cure was blood-letting, which meant taking blood from the patient (**D**). Frequent wars during the Middle Ages meant that

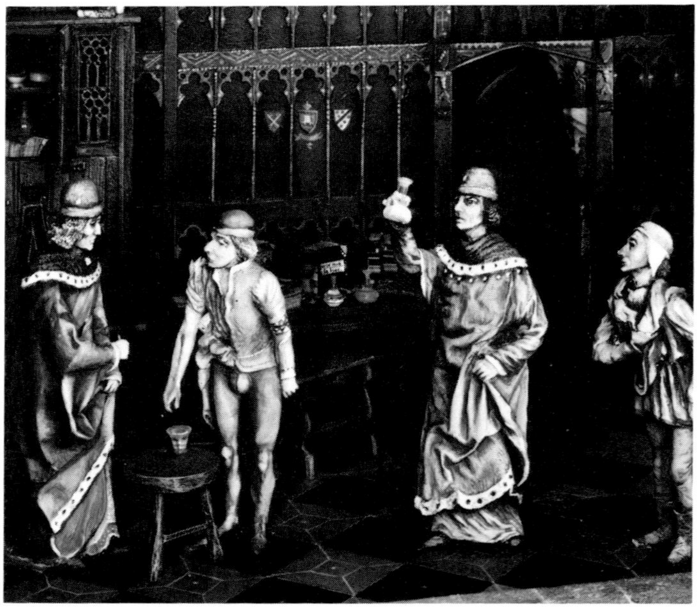

D A model of a medical consultation in the fifteenth century. The doctor on the extreme left is blood-letting the man next to him. The doctor standing second from the right is examining the urine of the patient on the extreme right.

E A 'zodiac man' chart from a physician's 'vademecum'

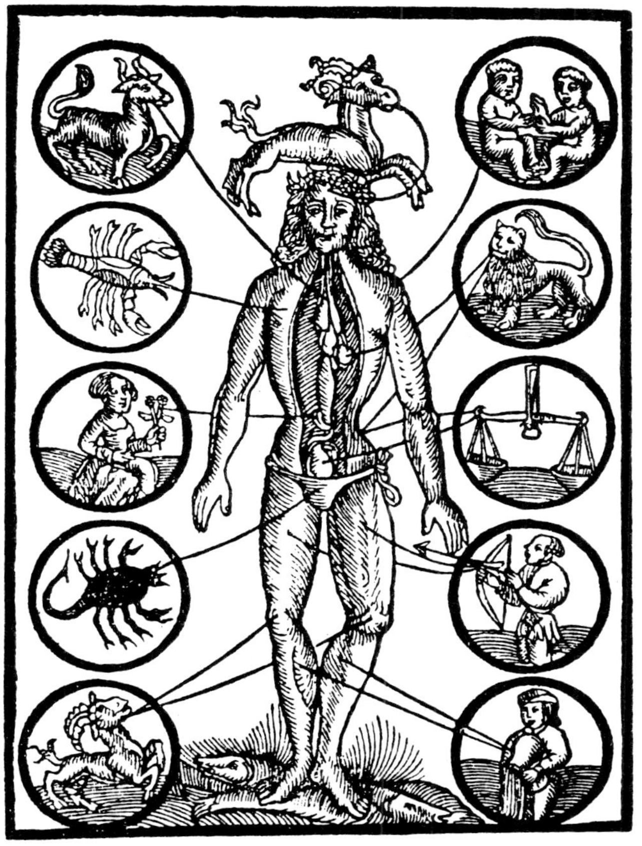

Aries	Avoid incisions in the head and face and cut no vein in the head.
Taurus	Avoid incisions in the neck and throat and cut no veins there.
Gemini	Avoid incisions in the shoulders and arms or hands and cut no vein.
Cancer	Avoid incisions in the breast and sides, stomach and lungs and cut no vein that goes to the spleen.
Leo	Avoid incisions of the nerves, lesions of sides and bones, and do not cut the back either by opening or bleeding.
Virgo	Avoid opening a wound in the belly and in internal parts.
Libra	Avoid opening wounds in the umbilicus and parts of the belly and do not open a vein in the back or do cupping.
Scorpio	Avoid cutting the testicles and anus.
Sagittarius	Avoid incisions in the thighs and fingers and do not cut blemishes or growths.
Capricorn	Avoid cutting the knees or the veins and sinews in these places.
Aquarius	Avoid cutting the legs and places as far as the heels.
Pisces	Avoid cutting the feet.

some surgeons were able to practise. But they would not have learnt very much as they had to work so quickly and in such bad conditions. Surgery was not taught in most medical schools. (Salerno, chapter 10, was the exception). In any case, dissection of the human body was forbidden by the Christian church.

There were *some* things that doctors did or suggested which we might feel were more sensible or scientific. Doctors often carried *Vademecums* which were pocket reference books. Although they often contained supersititious ideas like **E,** they also had urine charts showing different colours or shades of urine. A doctor could check a patient's urine sample as in **D** and learn something about his state of health.

In general, however, the Middle Ages in Europe saw a halt in the progress of medical ideas. Doctors relied on old books by writers such as Galen. We now know these books contained many faults. Until doctors worked out that there were mistakes very little progress would be made. There seemed to be little desire to change or to challenge these old ideas. It was not until the Renaissance began in about 1500 (see chapter 14) that any great strides in medicine were made.

??????????????????

1 Look at **A:**

a What is the writer's opinion of doctors?
b What three things does he accuse doctors of doing?
c Does he give any real evidence to support his view?
d How trustworthy do you think this is as a source of evidence? Give reasons for your answer.
e In **B** what would support Petrarch's view of doctors?

2 Would the 'cures' for toothache, fever and headache be likely to work? Why do you think people continued to use these cures? How do you think you would feel if you tried them out?

3 What is happening in **C**? What does it show about surgery in the Middle Ages?

4 **a** **D** shows one form of surgery used in the Middle Ages. Explain in detail what this is, using information from the chapter.
b **D** also shows one method of diagnosis used in the Middle Ages. Explain what this is in detail, using information from the chapter.
c Is **D** a primary or secondary source? Explain your answer and say how useful you think **D** is as historical evidence.

13 Health and Hygiene in the Middle Ages

Monasteries enjoyed a higher standard of hygiene than many other places during the Middle Ages. Some monasteries had lavatories (reredorters) and fresh water supplies from the rivers (**A**). Pictures like **B** show that people bathed and might therefore have seen the need to keep clean. Most ordinary peasants, however, shared their houses with their animals, and they very rarely washed themselves or their clothes. The women would boil scraps of meat fat to make a kind of soap to wash clothes. Water was often made softer by mixing it with

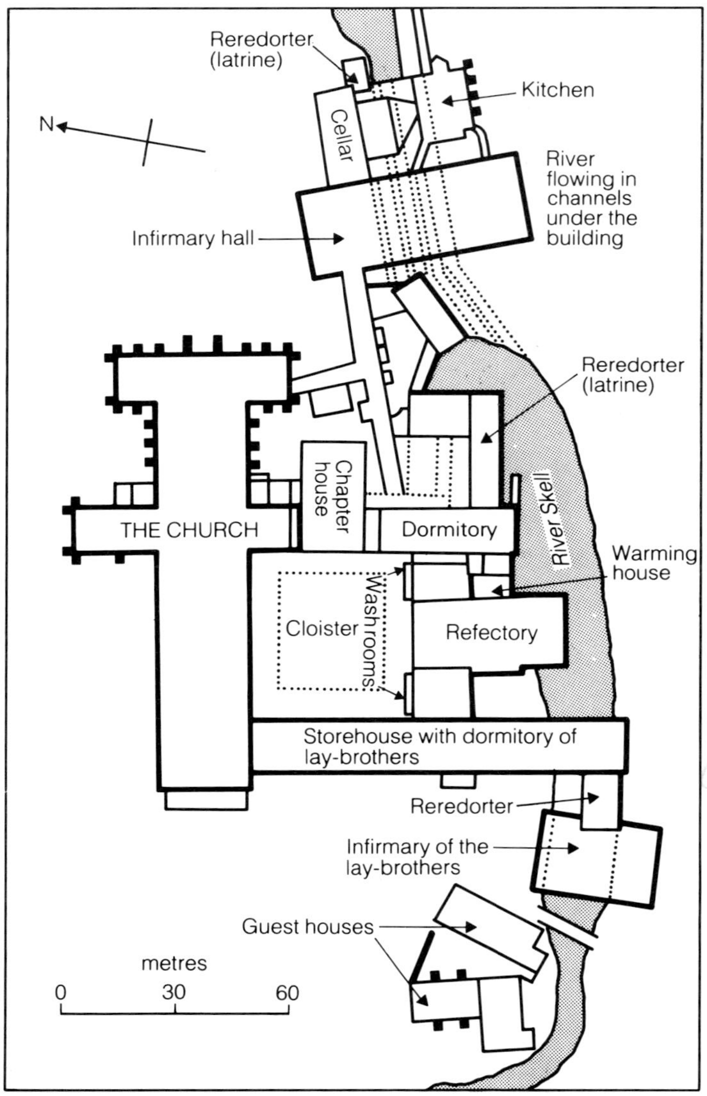

A A plan of the monastery at Fountains Abbey showing the existence of water supplies and drainage systems.

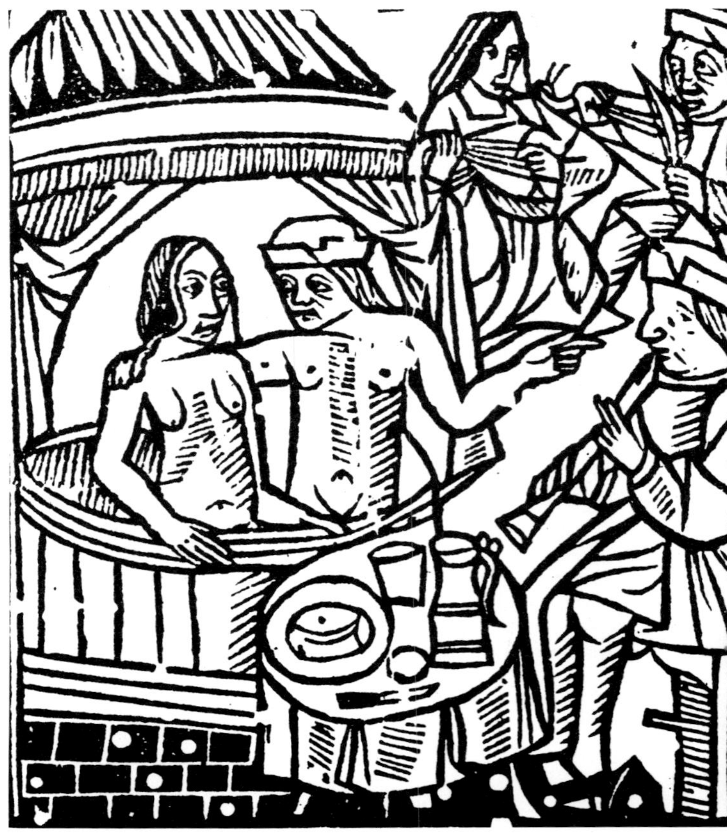

B A medieval woodcut of men and women bathing.

urine that had been stored in a jar for some months and the woollen industry used urine to treat their fibres. But people did not realize that they could avoid disease by keeping clean. A Dutchman, Erasmus, described a home he visited in 1518:

❛ *The floors are generally strewn with clay, and that covered with rushes that are now and then renewed, but not so as to disturb the foundation, which sometimes remains for about twenty years, nursing a collection of spittle, vomits, excrements of dogs and human beings, spilt beer and fishes' bones and other filth that I need not mention.* ❜ (**C**)

The streets of medieval towns were also very dirty. **D** shows a scene from a typical medieval town. The streets often had open sewers running down the middle of them. These sewers became clogged with rubbish and excrement thrown from the windows. Pigs, dogs and rats often roamed through the streets. Towns such as London sometimes tried to clean up the streets, but not very often.

People had no idea that dirty conditions could lead to disease. During the 1340s the Black Death (Plague) spread across Europe. It was a horrible disease, causing boils and fevers, and it killed more than a third of the people in less than ten years. We now know that the disease was caused by germ-carrying fleas that lived on the black rats which flourished in the dirty conditions in the streets all over Europe. At the time, however, people had other ideas about the cause of the disease:

❛ *The Death began at 1pm on 20 March 1345. Jupiter sucked up bad air and Mars spat it out. The great sea near India began to boil. Reptiles crawled out of the sea and spread the disease.* ❜ **(E)**

Guy de Chauillac, a physician trained at Salerno

❛ A priest: *The disease is sent from God as a punishment for our sins.*
A German man: *The Death is caused by the Jews who have poisoned the drinking water.* ❜ **(F)**

There were also flagellants who whipped themselves because they thought the disease was a punishment from God to make them suffer. Some cures included crouching over toilets and sniffing in the smell, taking *theriac* (a potion partly made up of the bodies of chopped up snakes that had been dead for ten years) and following the slogan *Fast Far Late,* which meant run as fast as you could, go as far away as you could and come back as late as possible.

Yet, there is evidence which shows that the people of the Middle Ages did have some idea of how to slow down the spread of diseases. Leprosy was almost wiped out by the end of the Middle Ages in Europe. Lepers were not allowed to touch the things they wanted to buy. They had to point at things with a stick. They had to shake a rattle to let people know they were coming. Towards the end of the period, lepers were isolated (kept apart) in special hospitals called *lazarettos.* There were more than 20 of these in France alone.

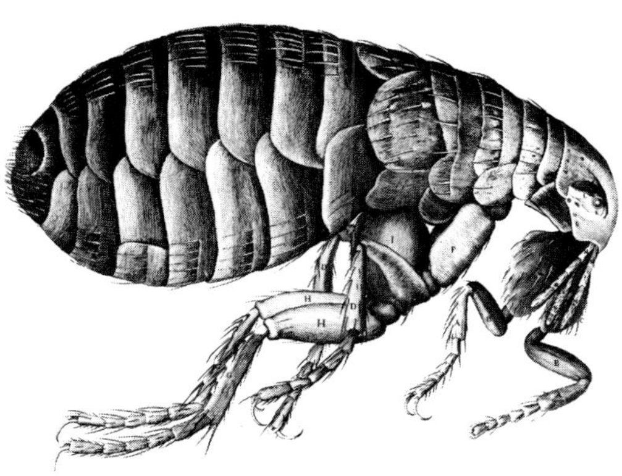

G A flea (enlarged many times)

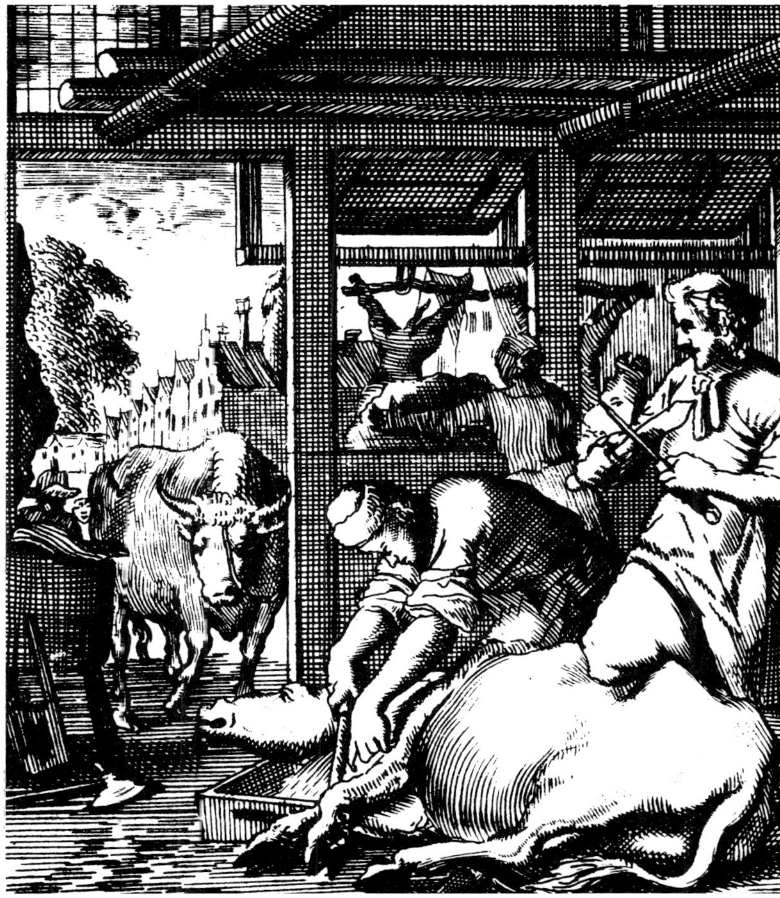

D A slaughter house in a medieval town

??????????????????

1 If you were a doctor or a health visitor visiting **D** what would you put in your report about the health hazards?

2 a What do **A** and **B** tell us about hygiene in the Middle Ages?
b Do sources **C** and **D** contradict what **A** and **B** suggest? Give reasons for your answer.

3 What do **C, D, E** and **F** tell us about what people knew of the causes of disease during the Middle Ages?

4 List three things done to control leprosy and explain how each one would have helped to stop the disease from spreading.

5 Use all the information in the chapter to explain how you think the Black Death spread so quickly throughout Europe. Mention streets, houses, people's actions, ideas about causes and remedies tried.

14 The Renaissance 1500-1700

During the sixteenth century, a rebirth (Renaissance) took place in learning in Europe. Progress in medicine and many other areas was very fast. The invention of the printing press in the fifteenth century was one of the main aids to the spread of learning in the Renaissance. Re-edited Greek medical books were printed. Physicians began to study them with great care and challenge some of their ideas.

Voyagers like Christopher Columbus discovered and explored new lands and brought back to Europe new ideas, herbs, plants and medicines. Monardes, a Spaniard, wrote the first book about the healing properties of plants which the Spanish sent back after 1520 from their newly found and conquered lands in the New World – Central and South America.

Changes in art also helped medical knowledge. Artists like Michelangelo, the painter of **A,** studied and drew the body in precise detail. This helped surgeons by providing drawings in books on surgery. The study of anatomy began again and the cutting up or dissection of human corpses took place in anatomical theatres like **B.**

For more than a thousand years most Europeans had accepted the mistaken teachings of writers such as Galen. Can you remember why they believed him? But, between about 1500 and 1700, thinkers and teachers in universities began to challenge many of the old ideas and put forward new ones of their own.

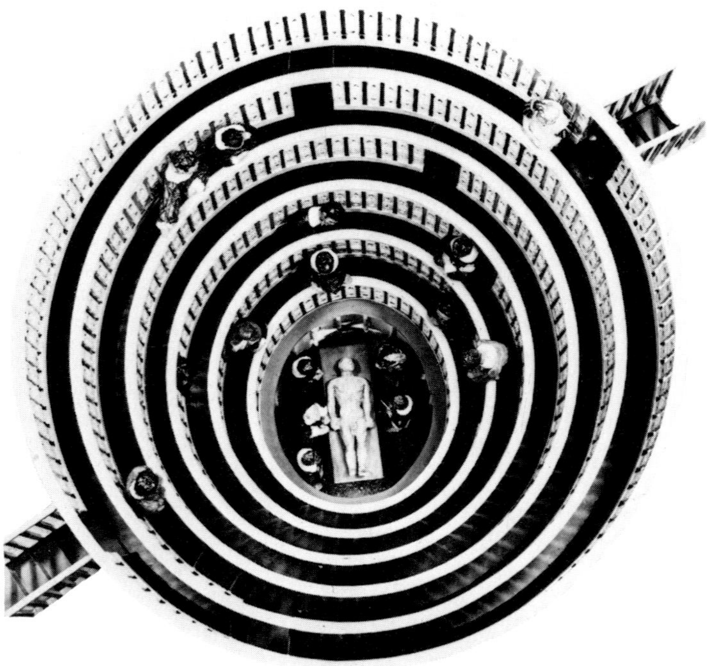

B A model of the anatomical theatre at the university of Padua in 1594. The theatre could hold 300 people, none of them more than 30 feet away from the dissection table.

A Some Renaissance artists practised dissection in order to be able to draw the human body accurately. This picture is from 'The Creation of Adam' by Michelangelo painted between 1508 and 1512.

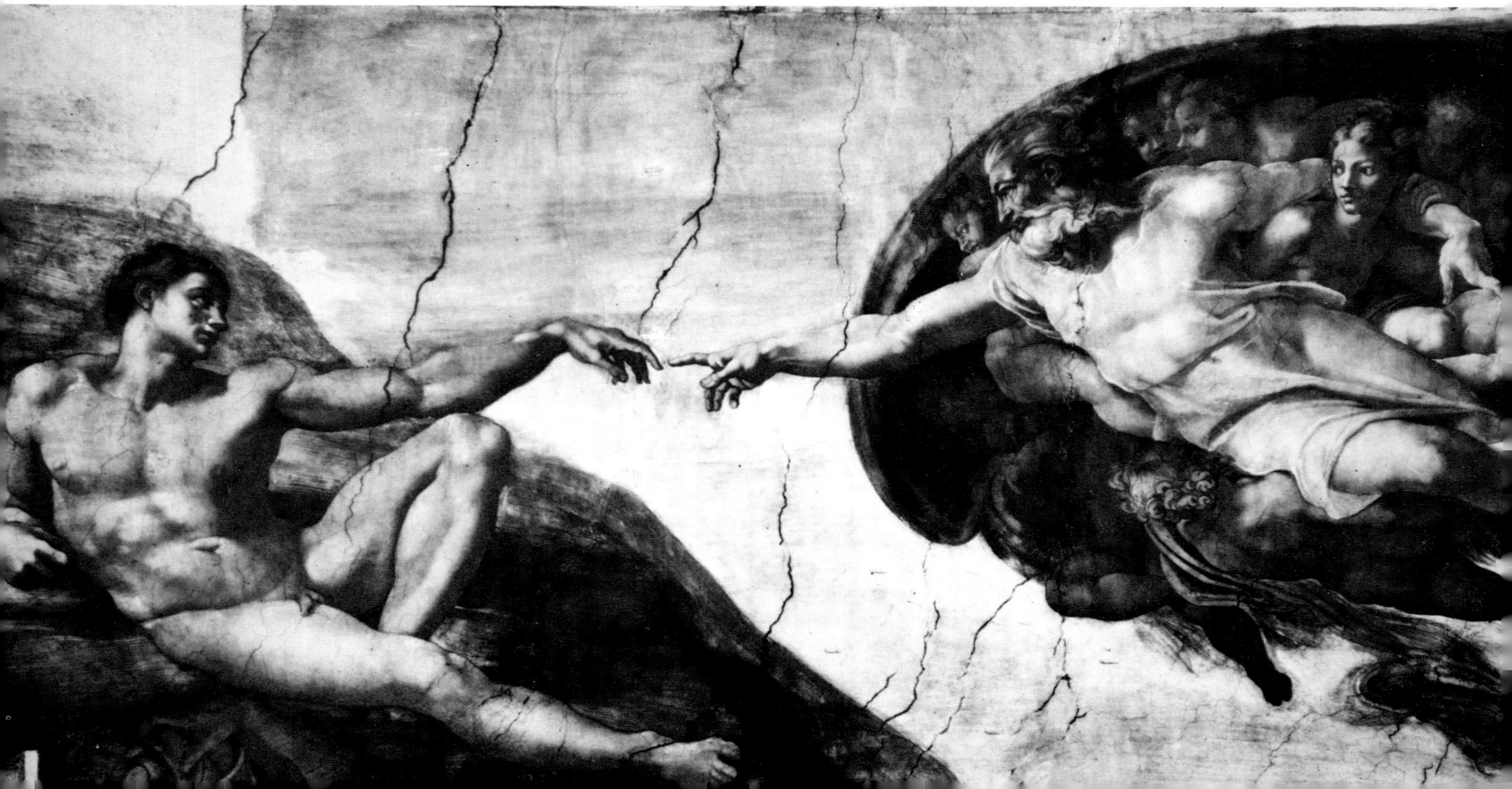

Paracelsus (1493-1541)

Aureolus Philippus Theophrastus Bombastus von Hohenheim, known as Paracelsus, is an example of a typical Renaissance man. He challenged existing ideas and put forward new ones. In 1523 he became a lecturer in Basel, Switzerland. The first thing he did before he lectured was to burn the books of Galen and Avicenna. He said to the students:

❛ *Galen is a liar and a fake; Avicenna is a kitchen master. They are good for nothing. You will not need them. Reading never made a physician. Patients are the only books. You shall follow me. I shall be the monarch of medicine.* ❜ (**C**)

He made men question medical ideas and look for answers for themselves. He insisted on observation and experience and used drugs and chemicals like laudanum, mercury, iron and sulphur. He is said to have told his students when treating a lunatic:

The doctor must tread nature's book with his feet. You should treat the spirit for it is the spirit that here lies sick. It is a major achievement to understand the ravings of the lunatic.

Many doctors rejected his ideas – can you think why? Only 200 years later did people begin to realize the value of his work.

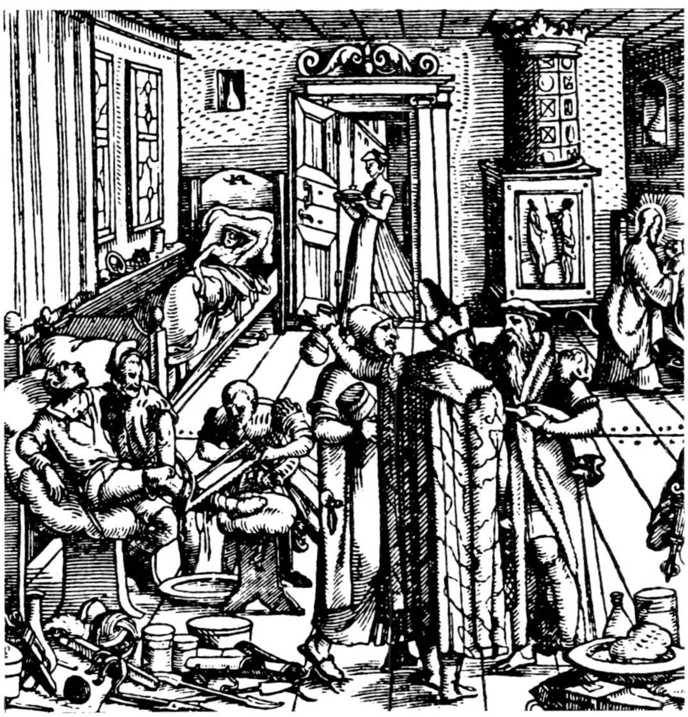

D From Paracelsus's book *Opus Chirurgium* – on the left an amputation is taking place and in the centre doctors are examining the urine sample of a patient.

Thomas Sydenham (1624-1689)

Thomas Sydenham was a famous London doctor who, like Paracelsus, thought that a doctor could learn most from looking at patients rather than books. He once told Hans Sloane (the founder of the British Museum): 'You must go to the bedside, it is there alone you can learn disease.' He believed in direct observation and this is why he is sometimes known as the English Hippocrates. He recorded the patient's progress, and suggested diet, rest and simple remedies.

Like Paracelsus, he was unpopular with the medical profession. But he was popular with his patients. The need for a good bedside manner and the ability to get on with people are stressed in medical schools today. Sydenham would certainly have approved of this.

??????????????????

1 Match the causes of change during the Renaissance in column A with the results they would bring in column B:

A Causes of change	**B Effects**
Voyagers discovered new lands such as America	Surgeons had to develop new techniques for treating wounds
The printing press was invented	Better anatomical drawings helped doctors and surgeons
Artists began to study the body in more detail	More people could learn from what had been learnt and written down in the past
New universities and schools grew up	Knowledge could be spread much more widely and quickly
The discovery of gunpowder	New foods and medicines, herbs and plants were brought back to Europe

2 In what ways did Renaissance art help medical knowledge? Refer to **A** and other information in the chapter to help you answer the question.

3 Look at **B** and **D.** Imagine you had visited the hospital and anatomical theatre shown. Write an account, of your visit.

4 a Why did Paracelsus burn the works of Galen and Avicenna?
b Which of Paracelsus's statements or achievements do you think is the most important? Say why.

5 Why is the term 'the English Hippocrates' a good one to describe Thomas Sydenham?

15 Vesalius, Paré and Harvey

During the Renaissance great thinkers in medicine made many discoveries which altered the way doctors and surgeons worked. Three such thinkers were Vesalius, Paré and Harvey.

Andreas Vesalius (1514-64)

Vesalius studied medicine at Paris. He learnt a lot by taking skeletons from the gallows. He would take the skeleton apart, soak the bones in vinegar to hide their decaying smell and smuggle them back into town to study.

A brilliant student, he became professor of anatomy at Padua University at the age of 23. Hundreds of students would pack the lecture theatre (see **B,** chapter 14) to hear him lecture. While other lecturers read aloud from the books of Galen and assistants carried out the dissections, Vesalius did the dissections himself. Vesalius, like Paracelsus, broke with the past when he told his students to study the human body for themselves instead of believing what they read in some of the old medical books by Greek and Muslim writers.

A Illustration from *The Fabric Of The Human Body* by Vesalius

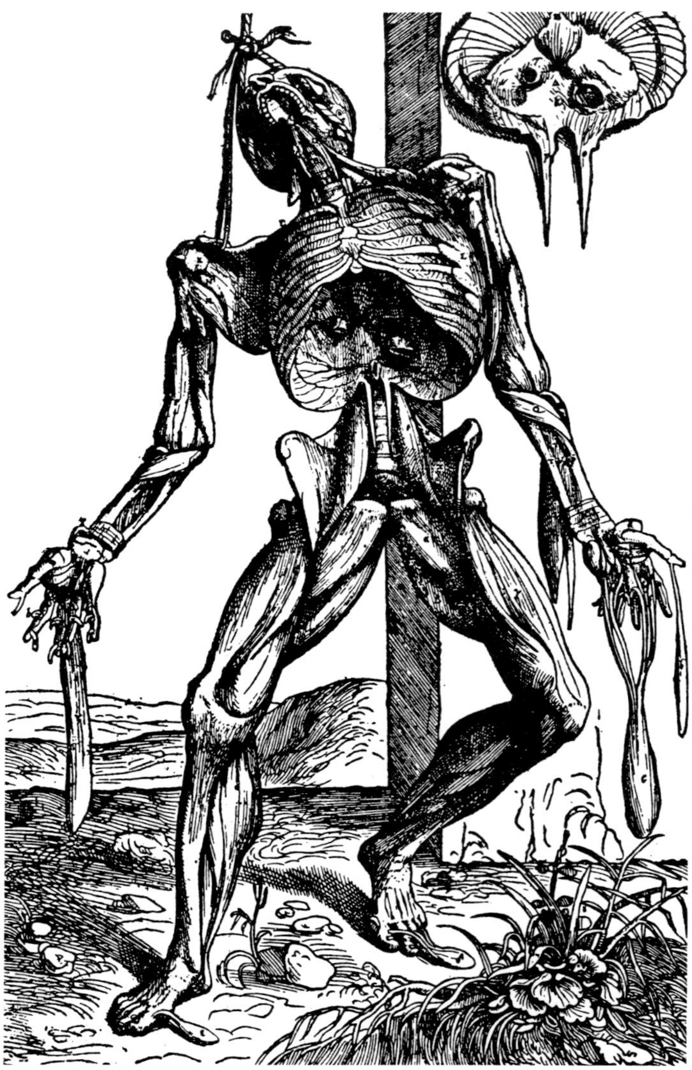

In 1543 he wrote a famous book, *The Fabric of the Human Body* (see **A**). Vesalius found out that Galen had made mistakes. Galen had said that humans had the same number of bones in the spine as the monkey. Vesalius discovered that this was wrong. He also found other mistakes, which he explained in the book.

❛ *The jaw of most animals is formed of two bones. In man, however, the lower jaw is formed of one single bone. Nevertheless, Galen and most of the skilled dissectors after the time of Hippocrates asserted that the jaw is not a single bone.* ❜ (**B**)

The older doctors and surgeons at Padua opposed Vesalius and made fun of his ideas. They may have been jealous of him because he had become successful while still a young man. But they were also angry that Vesalius had dared to suggest that Galen might be wrong. Partly because of these enemies Vesalius left Padua and worked as court physician to the Emperor Charles V. Vesalius's book and methods began a new era of progress in medicine.

Ambroise Paré (1510-1590)

Ambroise Paré changed people's ideas about surgery in the same way that Vesalius changed ideas about anatomy. He was helped by the large number of wars during his lifetime. In 1536 he joined the army as a barber-surgeon and spent the next 20 years on campaigns. **C** shows how gunshot wounds were treated before Paré. Wounds were cauterized with boiling oil as quickly as possible. The method was painful and very dangerous and the wounds often swelled afterwards. One day he was forced to try out a new method of healing a gunshot wound because the oil he was using had become too thick. He described what happened:

❛ *I applied in its place a digestive (ointment) made of the yolks of eggs, oil of roses and turpentine. That night I could not sleep at my ease, fearing by lack of cauterization that I should find the wounded dead or poisoned. Beyond my hope I found those upon whom I had put the digestive feeling a little pain and their wounds without inflammation (swelling). The others, to whom I had applied the boiling oil, I found feverish with*

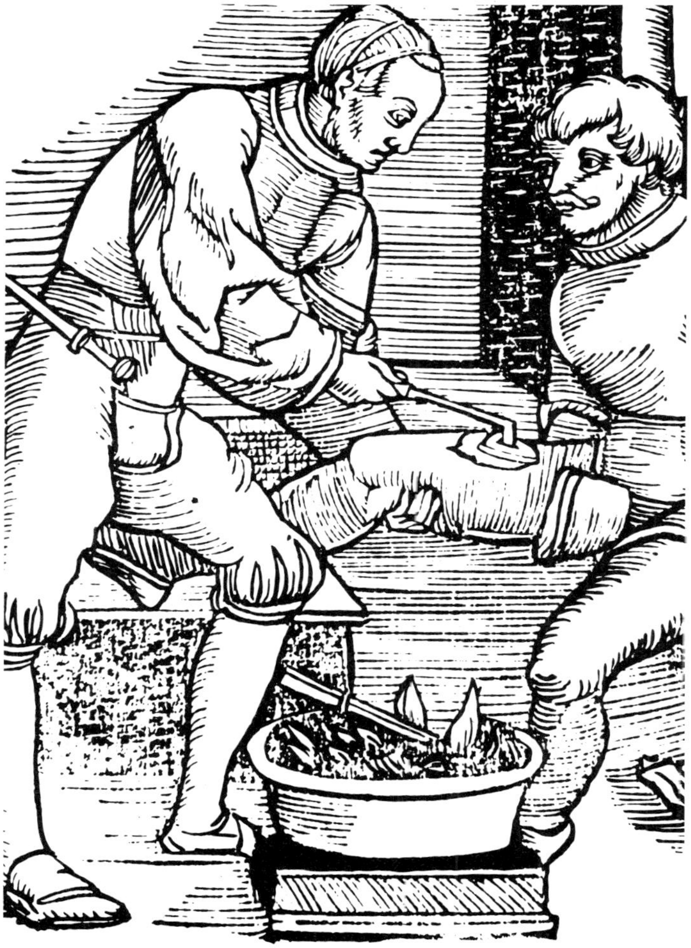

C A gunshot wound is cauterized (scorched with hot iron or boiling oil) to prevent infection.

great pain and swelling about their wounds. Then I resolved with myself never again to burn thus cruelly poor men wounded with gunshot. ❞ (**D**)

From The Apology and Treatise *by Ambroise Paré*

In 1575, Paré published *The Collected Works of Surgery* which had important effects on the treatment of wounds, amputations and the setting of fractures. Paré also made artificial limbs and new tools or instruments for surgeons to use.

William Harvey (1578-1657)

William Harvey (like Vesalius and Paré) relied on observation and experiment to increase his knowledge. By doing this he discovered that the heart pumps blood round the body in a continuous loop. **E** is a drawing from his book *An Anatomical Account of the Motion of the Heart and Blood in Mammals*. He used the drawing to explain an experiment he carried out to prove that the blood will travel only one way through the veins. He said that if the upper arm is bandaged (A), the valves (G,O,H) show up as nodules on the vein. If the finger is pushed along the vein from one valve to the next (e.g: B to C or C to D) away from the heart, the section of vein between the valves will be emptied of blood. It will stay empty until you take your finger off the valve.

Harvey's book increased people's understanding of how the body worked. He studied at most of the famous medical schools in Europe, including Padua where Vesalius had taught.

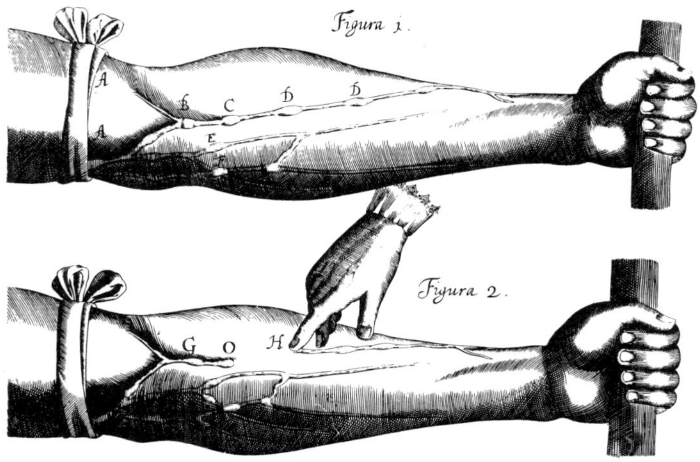

E A diagram of the veins of the arm to show that blood will travel only one way.

?????????????????

1 How would drawings like **A** have helped surgeons during the Renaissance?

2 Make a list, in order of importance, of five things that Vesalius did. Say why you put the first one at the top of the list and the last one at the bottom.

3 What did Vesalius say about Galen? How did Vesalius prove he was right and Galen wrong?

4 Imagine you are a soldier in the French army in the sixteenth century. Describe two different operations you have had for gunshot wounds, one before Paré joined the army, the other by Paré himself.

5 **E** is a diagram Harvey drew to explain an experiment he carried out.
- **a** What did the experiment prove?
- **b** What is the importance of Harvey's discovery?

6 How did each of the following affect Vesalius, Paré and Harvey?
- **a** The growth of universities
- **b** The invention of the printing press
- **c** The rebirth in art (work of artists)
- **d** Warfare

16 Medicine 1600-1800

A Medical discoveries and ideas	
Name	**Idea or development**
William Harvey (1578-1657)	Discovered the circulation of the blood by 1628.
Thomas Sydenham (1624-1689)	Began a new movement back towards the idea of Hippocrates that doctors could learn more from studying patients at the bedside than from books or study. He gave the first full accounts of scarlet fever, measles smallpox and gout.
Robert Boyle (1627-1691)	Showed by experiment that air was essential to life and disproved the idea that earth, fire, air and water were the four main elements.
Malpighi (1628-94)	Invented an efficient microscope that could be used to study blood.
King Charles II (1630-1685)	Founded Royal Society in 1661. It aimed to increase knowledge of nature by experiments and a more scientific approach to study. The Royal Touch came into fashion. Many people thought the King could cure them of the disease scrofula simply by touching them.
Stephen Hales (1637-1701)	The first person to measure blood pressure by inserting pipes into the arteries of animals.
Hermann Boerhaav (1668-1738)	Had a special ward where he used all the new aids for doctors that became available and put the new theories into practice. Students left his hospital in Holland and set up similar ones in France, Austria, Switzerland, England and Scotland.
Giovanni Morgagni (1682-1777)	Pioneered pathology or the study of how disease affects the human body
Albrecht Haller (1708-1777)	Studied and wrote about respiration, bone growth, digestion, muscles and nerves.
John Hunter (1728-1793)	Set up a school of surgery with his brother William in London in 1748.
Edward Jenner (1749-1823)	Discovered in 1796 that vaccination could be used to prevent smallpox.

Some of the developments in surgery and in aids for doctors during the seventeenth and eighteenth centuries are dealt with in detail in chapters 20 and 33. **A** summarizes the main discoveries and new ideas during this time.

Many people like those in **A** tried to take a more scientific approach to the study and practice of medicine. Yet their ideas were often opposed for many years before being accepted by doctors. It was not until the 1660s, for example, that most doctors believed William Harvey's views about the circulation of the blood. This was partly because Harvey's discovery meant that Galen was wrong. Most doctors at this time would not accept that Galen might be wrong. Malpighi was criticized throughout his life by his enemy Sparagli, who said that looking through microscopes and dissecting animals never helped to cure a single patient.

Why do you think people were so reluctant to accept new ideas? **B** might suggest an answer. It is from a modern history book and explains why people at that time often went on taking 'cures' for illnesses that we now know would have had no effect.

❛ *In medical treatment it must be realized that in acute illnesses particularly, such as fevers, the patient often recovers in the natural course of events, regardless of the treatment he is receiving. Few doctors, and even fewer patients, were content to attribute their recovery from serious fevers to this cause. Most would attribute their survival to the medicine they were receiving at the time of their improvement. In this way a vast number of 'cures' were achieved in practice. It is easy to understand how in those circumstances such medicines as crabs' eyes, powdered pearls and sheep's dung, acquired their reputation for curative properties.* ❜ **(B)**

From A Short History of Medicine *by Poynter and Keele*

C is some sentences from a book of remedies written in 1633. Do they show that beliefs about medicine had changed very much since the Middle Ages?

❛ *First consider what planet causeth the disease. Garden-Rue is an herb of the Sun, and under Leo the seed taken in wine is an antidote against all dangerous medicines. English tobacco is found by good experience to expel worms from the stomach when taken by a pipe, and the ashes of the burnt herb to cleanse the gums.* ❜ **(C)**

From Nicolas Culpepper's Complete Herbal *1633*

Royalty could not expect much better treatments than

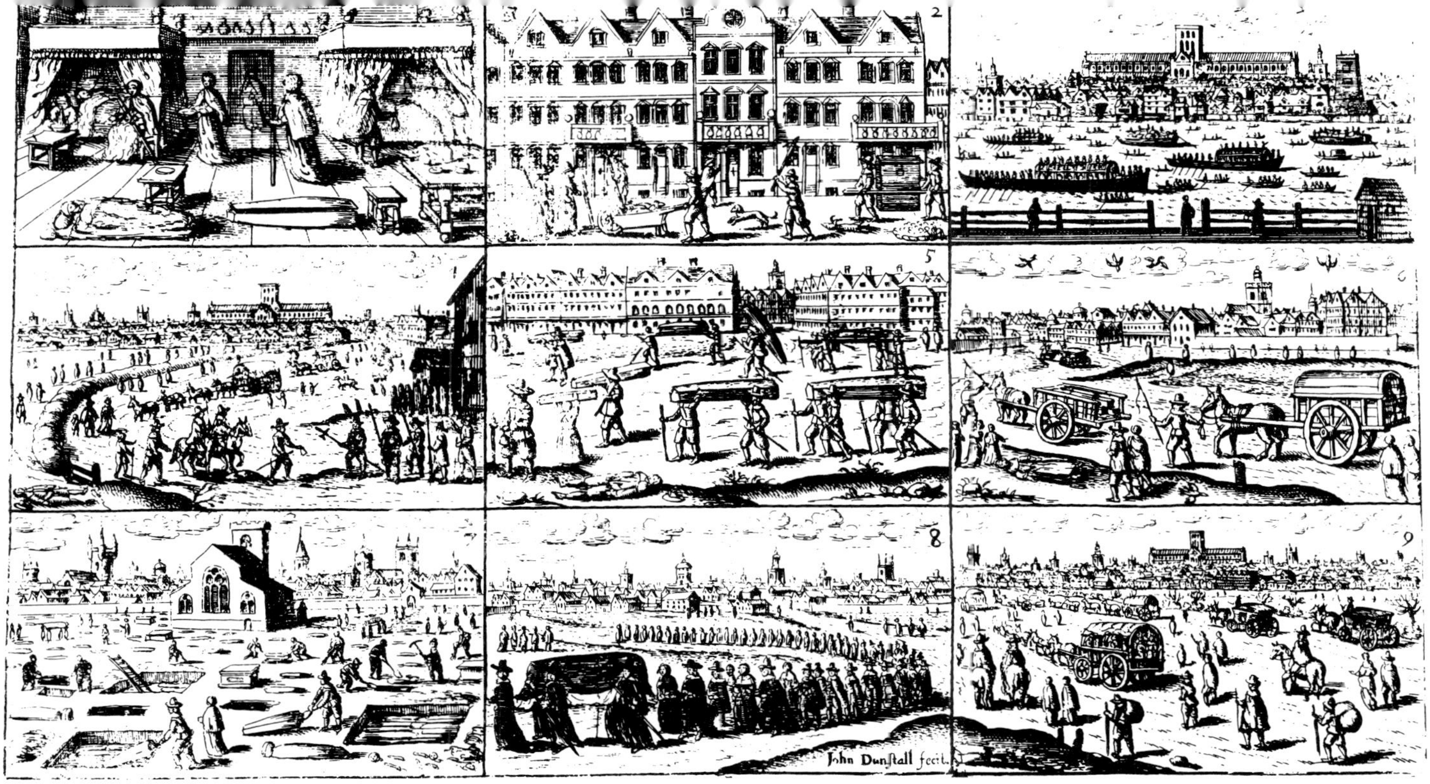

F A broadsheet showing scenes from the plague in 1665.

those shown in **C**. **D** shows some of the methods Charles II's doctors used to cure him of a fever before he died:

❛ *They opened a vein in his right arm and drew off about 16 ounces of blood . . . Within a few moments, so as to free his stomach of all impurities, they issued an emetic. Soon after, they gave one drachm of two-blend pills to drain away the humours. Over and above this, blistering agents were applied all over his head after his hair had been shaved.*❜ **(D)**

From Sir Charles Scarburgh's Account of the Death of Charles II

C and **D** show how doctors' knowledge of medicine had not grown a great deal since the Middle Ages. Many people were willing to accept superstitious beliefs about cures, as **E** shows:

❛ *His Majesty began to touch for the Evil according to custom, thus: His Majesy sitting under his state in the banqueting house, the chirurgeons cause the sick to be brought or led up to the throne where they kneel; the King strokes their faces or cheeks with both hands at once, at which instance a chaplain in his formality says; 'He put his hands upon them and healed them.' When they have been all touched they come up again in the same order and the other chaplain kneeling and having angel gold strung on white ribbons on his arms, delivers them one by one to his Majesty who puts them about the necks of the touched as they pass, while the chaplain repeats, 'This is the true light who came into the world.'*❜ **(E)**

From John Evelyn's diary, 1660

In 1665 another outbreak of the plague like the Black Death of 1348 (see chapter 13) broke out in London. **F** is an engraving from the time, showing some scenes during the plague and some of the actions that people took at the time. Do these actions suggest to you that people had learned anything about the cause of plague since the Black Death of 1348?

??????????????????

1 What do you understand by the phrase 'a more scientific approach to study'? Which people in **A** do you think were taking such an approach? Explain your answer.

2 **B** is a secondary source. Say,
- **a** why it is a secondary source
- **b** what point the author is trying to prove
- **c** where the author might have found his information
- **d** what other evidence in this chapter supports what the author is trying to say.

3 Imagine that you have an illness during the reign of Charles II. Describe the various remedies you take and why you take them. Refer to **C** and **D** and then describe your visit for the Royal Touch (see **E**).

4 Describe what actions people are taking in **F.** Put these actions into two columns, one column showing the actions that might help to control the disease and one column of actions that would not.

17 Jenner and Smallpox

In the late eighteenth and nineteenth centuries men like Edward Jenner and Louis Pasteur greatly advanced medicine.

Edward Jenner worked as a doctor in Chipping Sodbury near Bristol. He was told by a dairy maid that she would not catch smallpox because she had already had cowpox (a mild form of smallpox). In 1798 Jenner wrote:

❛ *It commonly happens that the disease is communicated to the cows, and from the cows to the dairymaids. Inflamed spots begin to appear on different parts of the hands. What makes the cowpox virus so extremely* unusual *is that the person who has been thus affected is forever after secure from the infection of smallpox.*

I selected a healthy boy, James Phipps, and matter from the sore of Sarah Nelme's hand was inserted on May 14th 1796 into the arm of the boy by means of two small cuts. *The same boy was inoculated the first of July with matter taken from a smallpox pustule, but no disease followed.* ❜ **(A)**

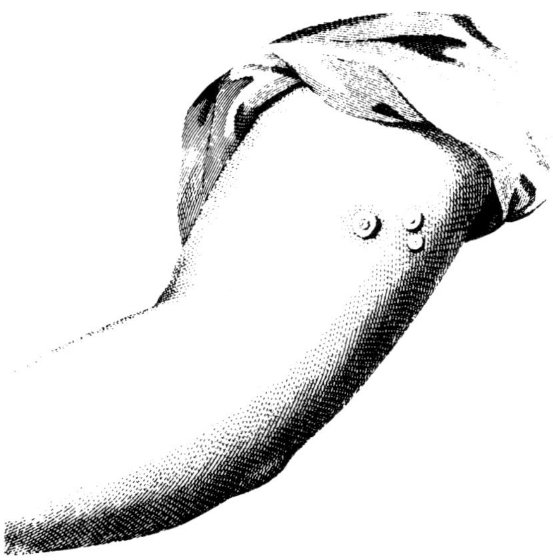

B Sarah Nelmes's arm showing cowpox sores.

Edward Jenner had discovered a cure for smallpox by using a method that has become known as *vaccination* (from the word *vacca* which is Latin for cow). But like many other men with new ideas, Jenner met opposition. In 1797 the Royal Society refused to believe his evidence and many others were not convinced (see **C**). It was not until 1802 that he was given a Government grant of £10,000 to develop his work.

In Jenner's time more than half the people of Europe would probably have had smallpox during their lifetime. Since 1977 there have been no recorded cases of smallpox. This is largely because vaccination (Jenner's discovery) eventually became compulsory in most countries.

This Day is published, Price One Shilling

A LETTER
from
JOHN BIRCH, Esq.

to the

EDITOR of the 'Fatal Effects of Cow Pox at Ringwood, Harlesden and other places.'

In this Publication are noticed
The Parliamentary Grant of £30,000 to Dr Jenner, for an unsuccessful Experiment;
A Letter, proving the Production of a new and fatal Appearance, called the

VACCINE ULCER

Described by Astley Cooper, Esq. Surgeon of Guy's Hospital
A Letter from Mr Westcott of Ringwood, proving the Failures of the Experiment at that Place;
A List of those who died of Cow Pox there;
A list of those who were defectively vaccinated and took Small-pox afterward; and of those who died of Small-pox after having been vaccinated, and assured of Protection;
A List of some Failures under the Treatment of the Vice President of the Jennerian Institution;

AND SEVERAL RECENT CASES

C An advertisement showing the letter from John Birch denouncing Jenner's vaccination.

??????????????????

1 a What is John Birch saying in **C**?

b For what other reasons might people have opposed Jenner and his ideas?

2 In 1958 28 million people in the world suffered from smallpox. In 1967 the figure was 10 million. Since 1977 there have been no recorded cases.

a Write an explanation of how smallpox has been eradicated (got rid of). Mention: vaccination, government grant to Jenner, compulsory vaccination.

b Why do you think so much time passed between Jenner's discovery of smallpox vaccination and the eventual eradication of the disease? What does this tell you about the speed at which new ideas in medicine spread?

18 Pasteur and Microbes

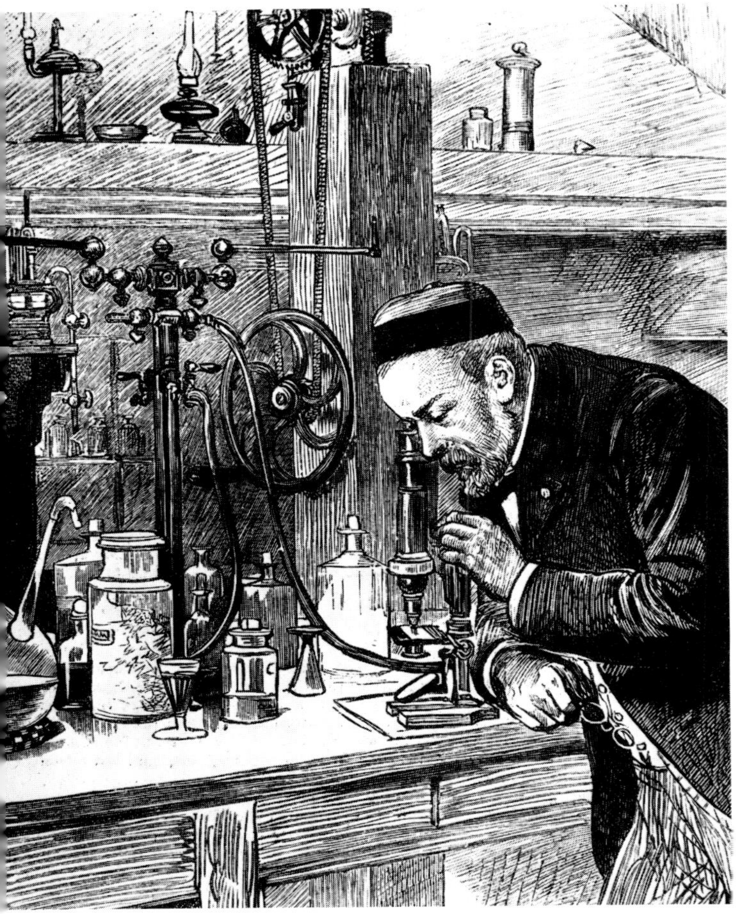

A Pasteur in his laboratory

Think of the pasteurized milk many people pour on to their cereal every morning. How does it get its name? The word comes from the name of Louis Pasteur (1822-95), a French chemist. The French wine industry asked him to find out why some of their wine kept going bad. With the aid of a microscope (see **A**), he saw microbes or tiny bacteria in the wine and realized that these might be causing its decay. He discovered that the germs died when he boiled the wine. The wine no longer went bad – it had been pasteurized. At the time most doctors believed that germs were caused by 'spontaneous generation'. This meant, for example, that the germs grew out of wounds and not that they came to the wounds from the air itself. Pasteur carried out an experiment that proved this wrong:

❛ *In a glass flask I placed . . . liquids that are extremely alterable through contact with ordinary air . . . I drew out the neck of the flask under a flame. I then boiled the liquid. The flask was then allowed to cool. The liquid treated in this manner remains indefinitely without alteration. The entrance of air slows down enough so that the dust it carries . . . is deposited on the moist wall of the curved tube. If, after one or two months, the neck of the flask is removed, moulds and germs begin to appear after 24, 36, or 48 hours just as usual.* ❜(**B**)

Pasteur had shown that germs causing decay are in the air all the time. His discovery was vital to the development of antiseptic surgery (see chapter 22).

Pasteur also isolated (sorted out) many bacteria that cause diseases. As a result of his work scientists developed *serums* (extracts from the blood of a person with a particular disease, which would be used for vaccination) to prevent anthrax and chicken cholera. In 1881 Pasteur developed a serum to stop people catching rabies. He became so famous, and his country was so grateful for his work, that in 1888 the French government built the Pasteur Institute in his honour. Here he went on teaching others until he died in 1895. Robert Koch, the bacteriologist, (see chapter 30) was one of his pupils.

C Pasteur's Discoveries

1 Proved that fermentation in wine was the result of the presence of micro-organisms which also caused decay.

2 Discovered how to eliminate germs from liquids (pasteurize).

3 Used Edward Jenner's practice of vaccination to stop anthrax, after isolating the bacillus which caused it.

4 Prepared vaccinations for chicken cholera, diphtheria and later for rabies (hydrophobia). The death rate from rabies (which had always been fatal) was reduced to less than 1 per cent by Pasteur's discovery.

??????????????????

1 Explain how each of the following was helpful to Pasteur: the microscope, the French wine industry, the French government.

2 At Pasteur's seventieth birthday celebrations, the British surgeon Joseph Lister said of Pasteur, 'Truly there does not exist in the wide world an individual to whom medical science owes more'. From the evidence in this chapter, why do you think Lister said this?

19 The Industrial Revolution

A Advances in medicine and public health after the Industrial Revolution

1847 James Simpson uses chloroform as an anaesthetic
1848 First Public Health Act
1859 Medical Register established – first official list of doctors
1864 Louis Pasteur proves that disease is caused by bacteria
1865 Joseph Lister pioneers antiseptic surgery
1875 Second Public Health Act compels town councils to make provision for water supply, sewage disposal and drainage
1882 Robert Koch isolates bacteria that cause TB and cholera
1895 Aspirin replaces opium as the major pain killer
1902 Midwives Act – Midwives to be registered and to receive special training.

Do you think that, in the 12000 years of history covered so far in this book, man had made much progress in medicine? If not, why not? **A** shows that between 1847 and 1902 many changes took place in medicine. Why did these changes suddenly take place? One reason was the great increase in scientific knowledge during the Industrial Revolution. Doctors and surgeons were able to use the discoveries of science to help treat patients and cure disease. Another reason was that changes in industry meant surgeons could invent complex machines to carry out new kinds of operations.

Medicine and public health needed to change because of the great increase in population in Britain during the nineteenth century (see **B** and **C**), and the rise of large, squalid industrial towns. **D** gives you an idea of what life was like in one of these cities – Manchester, a cotton spinning centre. **E** and **F** give us an idea of what jobs people did. Many people lived in cramped and dirty homes where diseases easily spread.

Solutions needed to be found for the problems that the *Industrial Revolution* (the growth of industry between 1780 and 1850) brought about. **A** shows some of the ways people tried to solve these problems. Much of the rest of this book deals with the effects of the Industrial Revolution.

B The increase in population

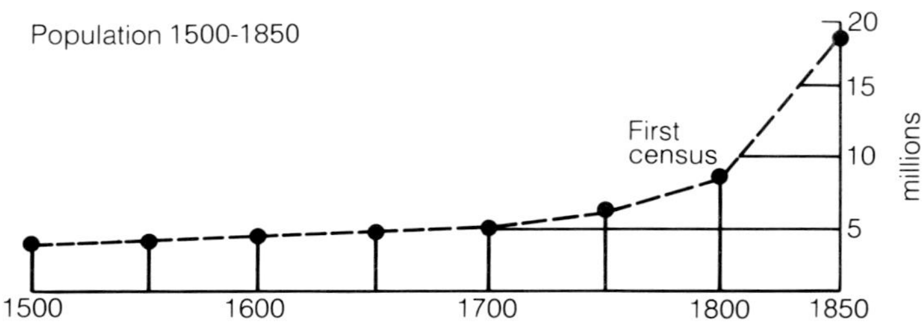

C The drift to the big cities

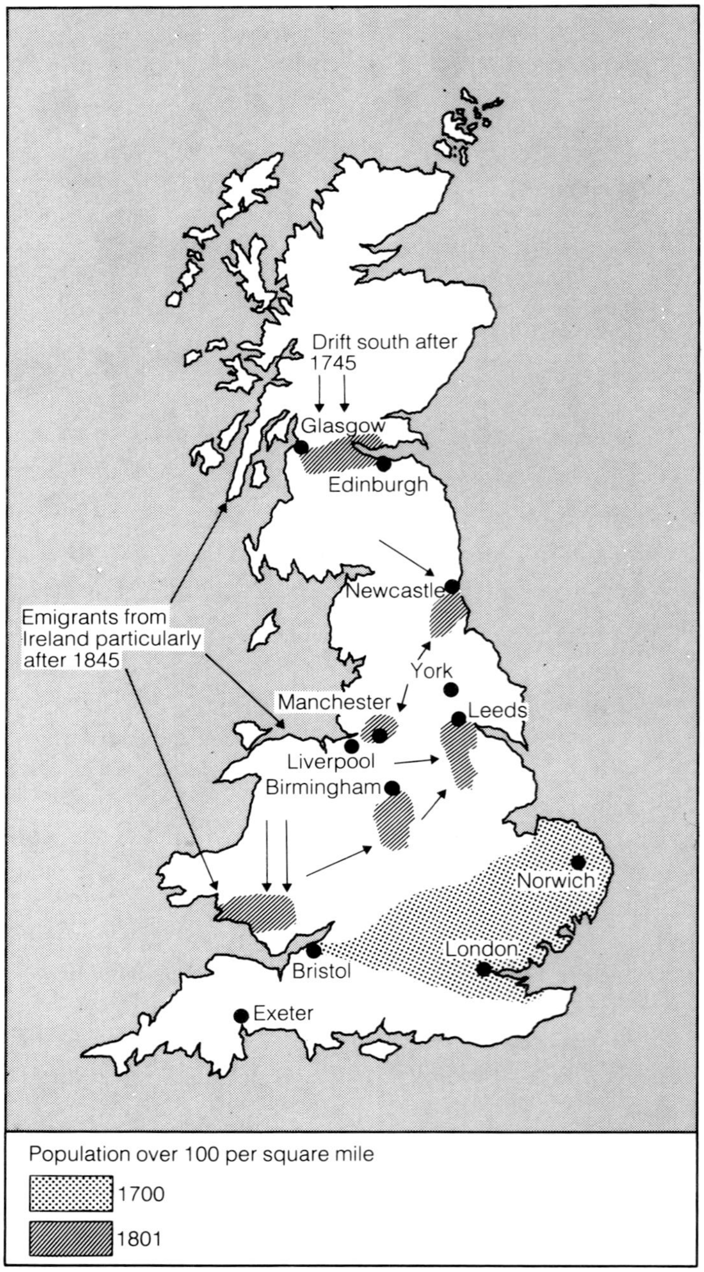

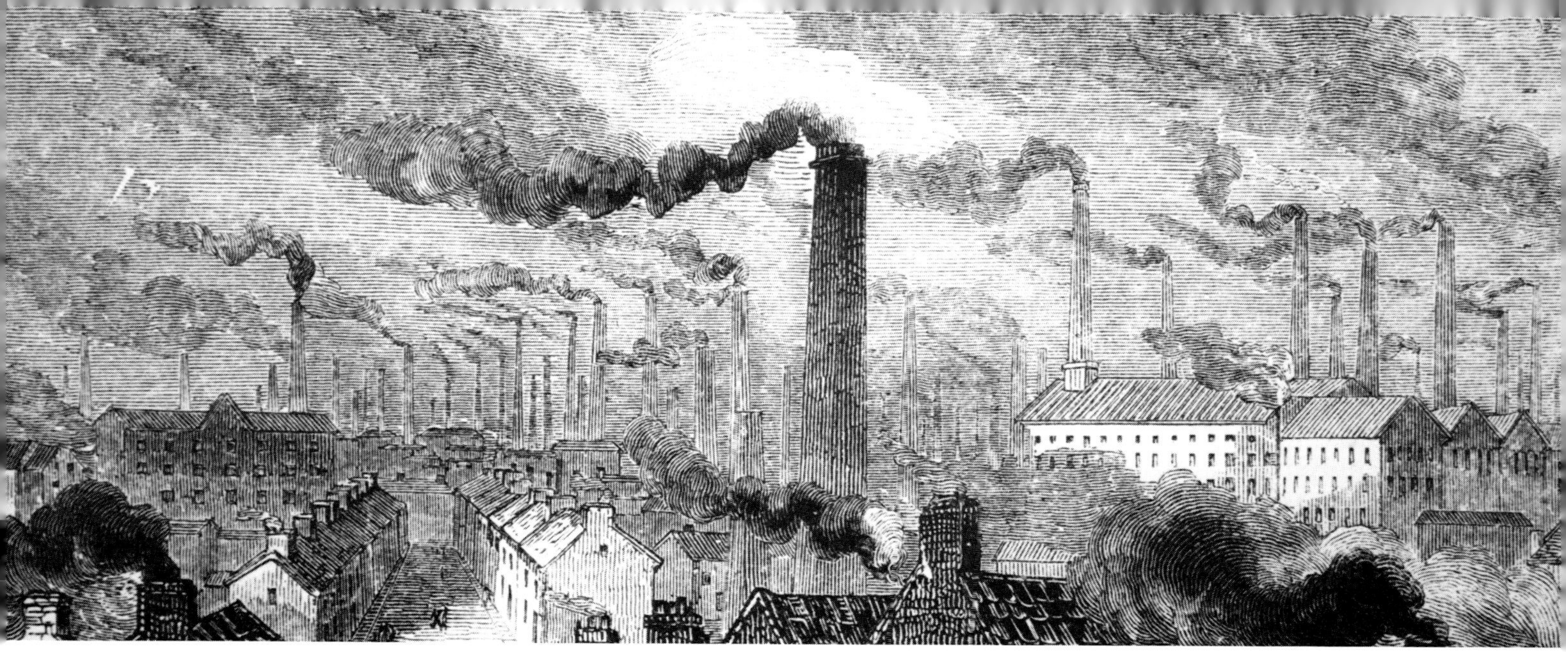

D Manchester in 1850

Main Jobs in 1688		Main jobs in 1851	
Labourers and servants	1,092,000	Farmworkers	1,790,000
Farmworkers	990,000	Domestic servants	1,039,000
Craftsmen	180,000	Textile workers	527,000
Seamen	150,000	Building workers	443,000
Shopkeepers and traders	120,000	Labourers	376,000
Gentlemen (landowners)	36,000	Sewing women	340,000
Merchants	30,000	Wool workers	284,000
Clergymen (vicars, priests)	30,000	Shoemakers	274,000
Government officials	20,000	Coalminers	219,000
Lawyers	20,000	Tailors	143,000
urce: Gregory King, an economist 10 wrote at the time		*Source:* 1851 Government census	

hanges in jobs

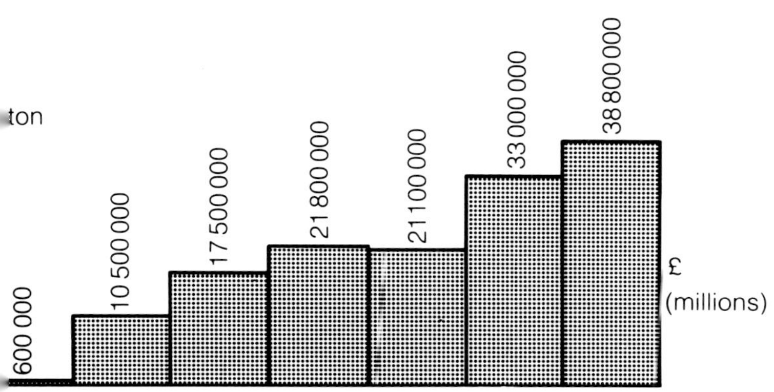

The increase in the textile industry

?????????????????

1 Put the list of achievements shown in **A** into what you think is their order of importance. Explain why you put the first one first and the last one last.

2 Rewrite the following paragraph, filling in the missing words: The Industrial Revolution (1780——) had a great effect on the progress of medicine. Between 1800 and 1850 the population of England and Wales rose from —— to ——. In 1700 most people had worked as farmers. By 1851 the third most popular occupation was ——. Factories were built in towns such as (list three towns shown in **C**) ——. Overcrowding and poor living conditions in the towns meant that many people died of diseases such as ——.

3 If you had had to live in the town in **D** during the 1850s, what would it have been like? Tick the most likely answers:

Healthy	Unhealthy
Clean Homes	Dirty homes
Smoky	Clean Air
Dirty Streets	Clean Streets
Crowded Homes	Uncrowded homes
Water, gas	No water, gas
Doctors	No doctors
Schools	No schools
Parks, playing fields	No parks, playing fields
Happy people	Unhappy people

What does this suggest about health in the 1850s?

4 In what ways did the problems caused by the Industrial Revolution affect the progress of medicine?

20 Developments in Surgery

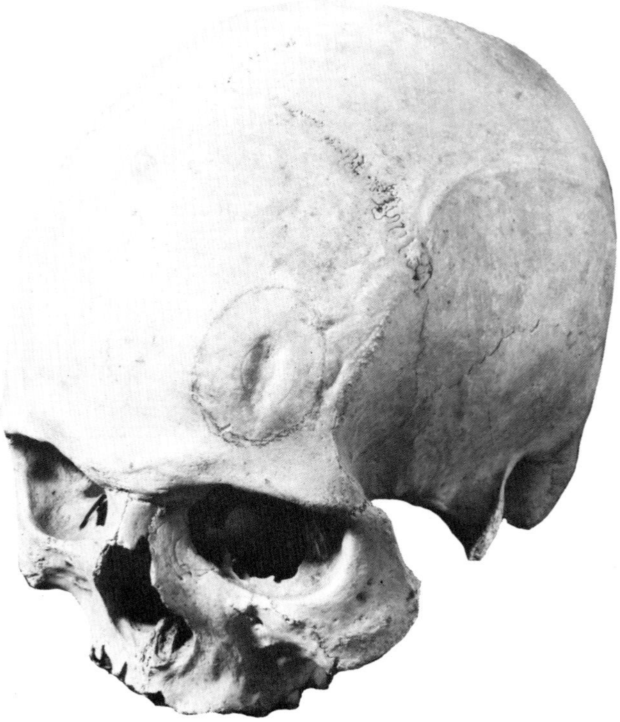

A A trepanned skull

The skills of surgeons had not improved very much by 1800. **A** shows that surgical operations date from prehistoric times. **B** is of ancient Egyptian surgical instruments and we also know that the Romans had surgeons who operated on soldiers. But, even as late as the sixteenth century, techniques in surgery were very primitive compared to those of today. Ambroise Paré, the army surgeon who did so much for the treatment of wounds in the sixteenth century (see chapter 15), realized how limited his surgery still was when he wrote:

❛ *We entered pell-mell into the city . . . and in a stable found four dead soldiers and three propped against a wall . . . They neither saw, heard nor spoke and their clothes were still smouldering, burned with gunpowder. As I was looking at them with pity there came an old soldier who asked me if there was any way to cure them. I said no. Then he went up to them and cut their throats gently and without ill will.* ❜ (**C**)

You may still see a red and white pole outside a barber's shop. The white stands for bandages and the red for blood. This is because before 1800 many operations were carried out by barber-surgeons (**D**). These untrained barber-surgeons were looked down on by the physicians (doctors) who had been to medical schools. Most people who studied medicine did not study surgery because it was not thought to be a true part of medicine. This was largely because of the work of barber-surgeons.

Surgery only became a branch of medicine when surgeons other than barbers practised in hospitals. This was due to the work of men such as William Cheselden (1688-1752). Cheselden was a surgeon at St Thomas's hospital in London. He became famous for carrying out successful operations. It was said that he could remove stones from the bladder in sixty seconds. Speed was very important in those days because there were no anaesthetics.

In Italy, during the 1750s, Giovanni Morgagni taught pathological anatomy for the first time. This is the study of disease – he dissected diseased corpses to find out about the spread of disease. From Morgagni's work doctors could learn exactly which organs of the body needed surgery.

B Egyptian surgical instruments from an original stone carving. These show that some surgery probably went on in Ancient Egypt despite the religious beliefs that the body was needed after death, which meant that dissection was forbidden.

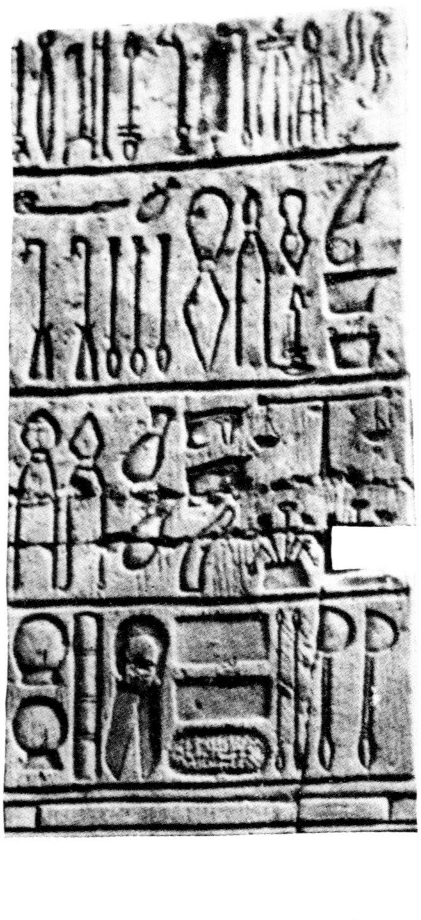

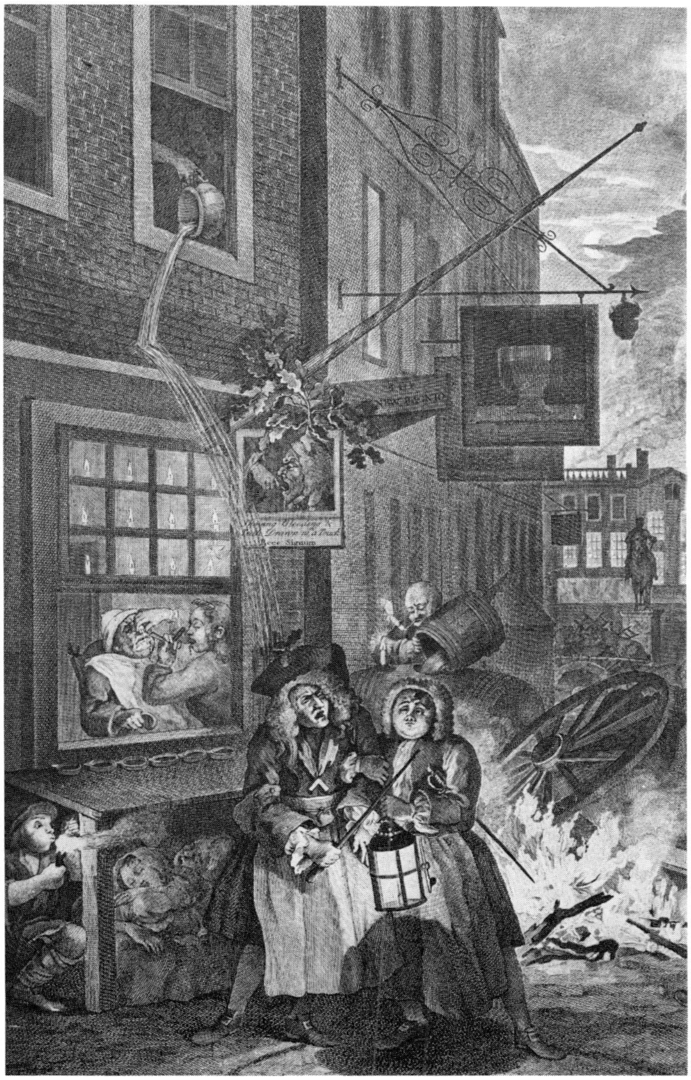

D A barber-surgeon's shop in the eighteenth century from a painting by Hogarth. The sign outside the shop says 'Shaving bleeding and teeth drawn with a touch'.

William Hunter set up a medical school in his own front room in Windmill Street in London where he taught surgery. In 1748 his brother John joined him as an assistant during dissections. John learnt quickly, studied surgery himself and began teaching others. They collected anatomical specimens so that others could learn about surgery.

In 1778 the Royal College of Surgeons of Edinburgh was set up. In 1784 and 1800 similar societies were set up in Ireland and London. These societies meant that surgeons had to register and could be taught properly. Surgeons could now gain proper qualifications. This was only the beginning of modern surgery and the next chapters will show how much the techniques of surgery have improved since the days of William and John Hunter.

??????????????????

1 Match up the heads and tails shown below:

HEADS

In prehistoric times . . .

In ancient Egypt, carvings showing surgical instruments have been found, which suggests that . . .

In Roman times . . .

During the Renaissance surgery had still not progressed very far as . . .

In the eighteenth century surgeons were looked down upon . . .

TAILS

we know that surgeons got some experience by working with soldiers on the battlefield.

the battlefield was still the main training ground for surgeons.

primitive surgery was carried out. Holes were drilled in skulls, perhaps to release demons.

because they were often barbers, not physicians.

some form of surgery was carried out, though it may have been done badly. The surgeon's knowledge of anatomy was limited, because religious beliefs did not allow dissection.

2 a What are the main disadvantages that an army surgeon had to face in the sixteenth century? Mention; speed at which they had to work, cleanliness, dangers, distractions, medical equipment, after-care.

b Can you think of any ways that warfare might have helped the development of surgery?

3 Imagine you are a student of surgery between 1745 and 1752. Write a diary in which you use and add to the following phrases:

4 June 1745: I saw William Cheselden perform an operation at St Thomas's hospital. He . . .

2 April 1751: I arrived in Italy and was told about the development of a new science (pathology). Giovanni Morgagni . . .

2 July 1752: I met William and John Hunter today. They have done so much to raise the standard of surgery in Britain. For instance . . .

21 The Discovery of Anaesthetics

While I was at the Edinburgh Infirmary I saw some operations under ether inhalations, a new method of rendering patients insensible to pain. A great blessing, but Professor Syme rather opposes it on account of the delay and the uncertainty as to the action of the ether, but the matter is still in its infancy.

Dr H. Cree, surgeon, January 1847

Although Cheselden and the Hunters had done much to improve the ways in which surgeons operated, it was only in the late 1840s that the problem of pain was first overcome. When you go for a operation today, you are first injected with barbiturates to put you to sleep. During the operation you are given an *anaesthetic* (something to relax the muscles and keep you asleep) which you breathe in through a mask. You feel no pain during the operation. We owe the discovery of anaesthetics to men like those in **A.**

B shows how a typical amputation would have taken place in the early nineteenth century. **C** describes an operation carried out by the surgeon Sir Robert Liston in December 1846. Imagine the pain you would have felt if you had had to undergo this operation without any anaesthetic to put you to sleep!

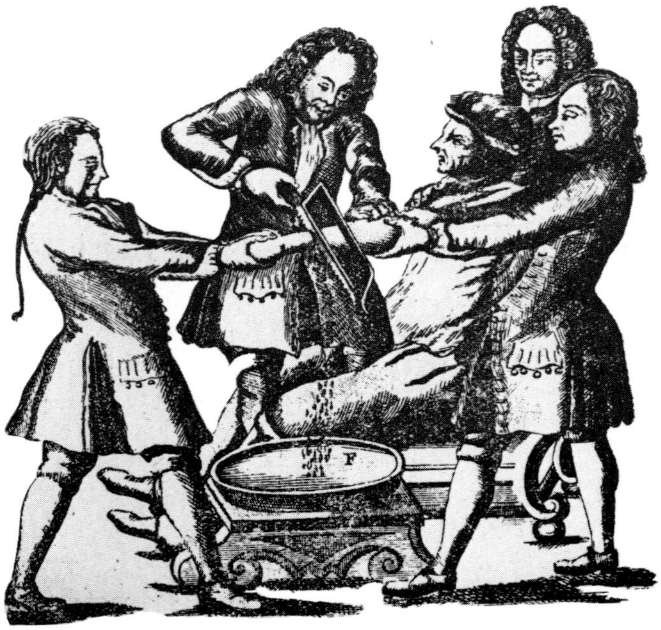

B An amputation in the early nineteenth century. Patients would be held firmly and told to bite hard on a piece of leather. They would often be blindfolded.

A

Person	Date	Anaesthetic	Details
Humphry Davy	1799	Nitrous Oxide (laughing gas)	Accidental discovery; eased pain but kept the patient laughing and conscious
Crawford Long	1842	Ether	Administered to a man having a tumour removed. Long did not publish the results of the experiment.
Horace Wells	1845	Nitrous Oxide	Used when extracting a tooth.
William Morton	1846	Ether	Used when extracting a tooth.
John Warren	1846	Ether	Removed a tumour at a public operation in Massachusetts.
Robert Liston	1846	Ether	Used to amputate a leg only three days after he had heard the news about Morton and Warren using ether.
James Young Simpson	1847	Ether	Used to help mothers during childbirth, although he found it did not work very well for this.
James Young Simpson	1847	Chloroform	After trial and error he discovered that chloroform was a better anaesthetic than ether.

❛ *He* (Liston) *then takes from his long, narrow case one of the straight amputating knives of his own invention. It is evidently a favourite instrument, for on the handle are little notches showing the number of times he had used it before. His house-surgeon, Ransome, puts the saw and the artery forceps on to the chair close by, then threads a wisp of well-waxed hemp ligatures through his own buttonhole . . . The porters are waiting just outside, and the patient is carried in on a stretcher and laid on the table . . . Liston stands by, trying the edge of his knife against his thumb nail, and the tension increases . . . Ransome holds the limb. 'Now, gentlemen, time me,' says Liston to the students. The huge left hand grasps the thigh, a thrust of the long, straight knife, two or three rapid sawing movement and the upper flap* (of skin) *is made. Half a dozen strokes and Ransome places the limb in the sawdust. 'Twenty-eight seconds!' says William Squires. The femoral artery is tied with two stout ligatures, a strip of wet lint placed between the flaps and the stump raised.* ❜ **(C)**

This is in fact an account of an operation carried out by Liston in 1846 in which he used ether as an anaesthetic

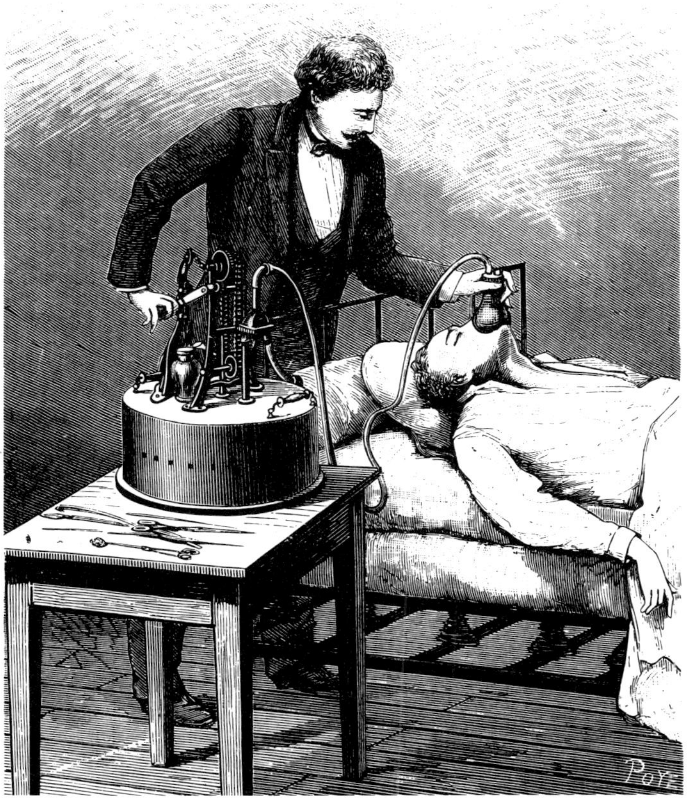

D This is how chloroform was inhaled in the late nineteenth century.

(see **A**). The patient felt no pain. If the operation had been carried out three days earlier (before Liston had heard of the use of ether), then the man would have suffered tremendous pain.

A shows how people experimented with various anaesthetics over a period of about 50 years. But it was not until 1847 that James Young Simpson discovered that chloroform was a more successful anaesthetic than any of the others. He used a rather dangerous and unscientific method to discover this. He and two of his friends simply sniffed different chemicals to see which ones would ease pain or put them to sleep. Eventually they stumbled on chloroform as a useful anaesthetic.

No one would doubt today the usefulness of anaesthetics. They have meant that longer and more complicated operations can be carried out more safely and without the patient feeling pain. It seems surprising therefore that the use of anaesthetics should ever have been opposed. But their use was opposed. Some doctors thought that the demonstrations of painless operations were 'staged' or 'fixed'. Some opposed anaesthetics on religious grounds, saying that, if God had not meant us to suffer, he would have made us in such a way that we would not feel pain. In 1853 much of the opposition to the use of chloroform as an anaesthetic disappeared. The reason is shown in this letter written to James Simpson:

❛ *The Queen had chloroform exhibited to her during her last confinement* (the birth of Leopold). *It acted admirably. Her Majesty was greatly pleased with the effect, and she certainly has had a better recovery. I know this information will please you, and I have little doubt that it will lead to a more general use of chloroform in the midwifery practice . . .* ❜ (**E**)

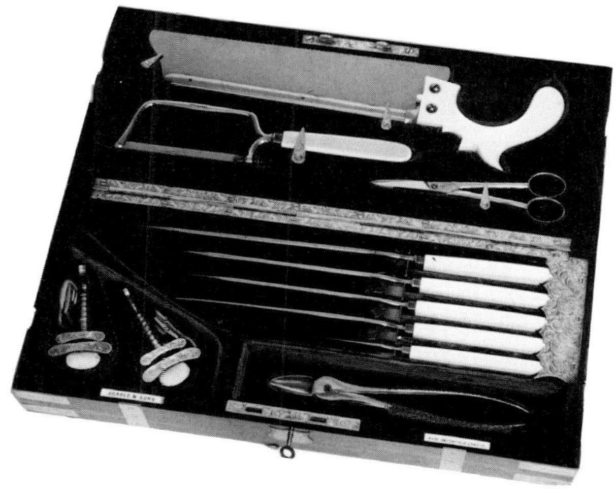

F A nineteenth-century amputation set

???????????????????

1 Complete the following paragraph by referring to **A**: The discovery of anaesthetics can be attributed to many men. In 1799 __________ accidentally discovered that laughing gas (N ____ O ______) relieved pain. ______ was used by Crawford Long in 18 ___ to remove a tumour. No one knew of Long's discovery, though, because ______ (complete the sentence). Three other people used ether as an anaesthetic. They were William Morton in 1846 ______ and ______ (name the others). But it was James Young Simpson in ______ who discovered that __________ was the most effective anaesthetic when used in childbirth.

2 Look at **B** and **C.** Describe how a typical amputation would be carried out before the discovery of anaesthetics.
Why do you think Liston had his operations timed?

3 Make drawings of three different surgical instruments shown in **F** and say what each one would have been used for.

4 Why would the information given in **E** be likely to 'lead to a more general use of chloroform in midwifery practice'?

22 Lister and Antiseptic Surgery

The discovery of anaesthetics (see chapter 21) meant that surgeons could carry out much longer operations and cut much deeper into the body of the patient. But, this meant there was more chance of the wound becoming infected. In Glasgow, for instance, in 1860 one third of the patients who had operations died afterwards from blood poisoning, which had spread from their wounds. Despite the ideas of Pasteur (see chapter 18), most doctors at the time thought that a poisonous mist in the air caused disease. Some patients thought that the dirtier a surgeon's coat was, the more operations he must have carried out, so, the greater the chance that they would survive if they let him operate on them.

❛*I remember the house-surgeon with his threaded needles dangling from the front of his coat, the silken threads sweeping the well-worn cloth which had grown old in the presence of sepsis* (blood poisoning). *One of our surgeons lectured on anatomy in an old frock coat. I see it now, faded with age, stained with blood and spotted with pus.*❜ (**A**)

Source **A** was written by someone who worked with Lister. What does **A** tell us about operations at this time?

In 1865, however, Joseph Lister (Professor of Surgery at Glasgow University) read Louis Pasteur's theory that disease was caused by bacteria. Lister, unlike many other doctors at the time, believed the theory and tried to do something to prevent patients from dying from blood poisoning in the hospital wards after an operation.

Lister tried many experiments that failed. Eventually he discovered that he could often prevent wounds from becoming infected by soaking bandages in carbolic acid and wrapping them around the wound. **B** shows the success of his methods in his treatment of fractures.

B	Years	Fractures treated	Recovered	Died
	1864-66	34	19	15
	1867-70	40	34	6

Lister then decided that the best way to prevent infection was to stop bacteria from getting to a wound in the first place. By the end of 1865 he was already insisting that bandages were used only once in his wards, that doctors and surgeons washed their hands regularly and that silk threads used for sewing up wounds were soaked in carbolic acid. His methods of trying to fight sepsis have become known as *antiseptic surgery* (**C** and **D**).

Because Lister was always willing to admit when he was wrong or when he thought his ideas could be improved, many people refused to accept his ideas and he was often made fun of. The writer of **E** suggests why.

❛*They* (other surgeons) *noted that Lister was constantly changing his techniques and came to the conclusion that this was because his results were not good. They apparently did not listen to the statement that he did so with the object of removing the irritation of the antiseptic* (caused by the carbolic spray).❜ (**E**)

C An operating theatre at the time of Lister

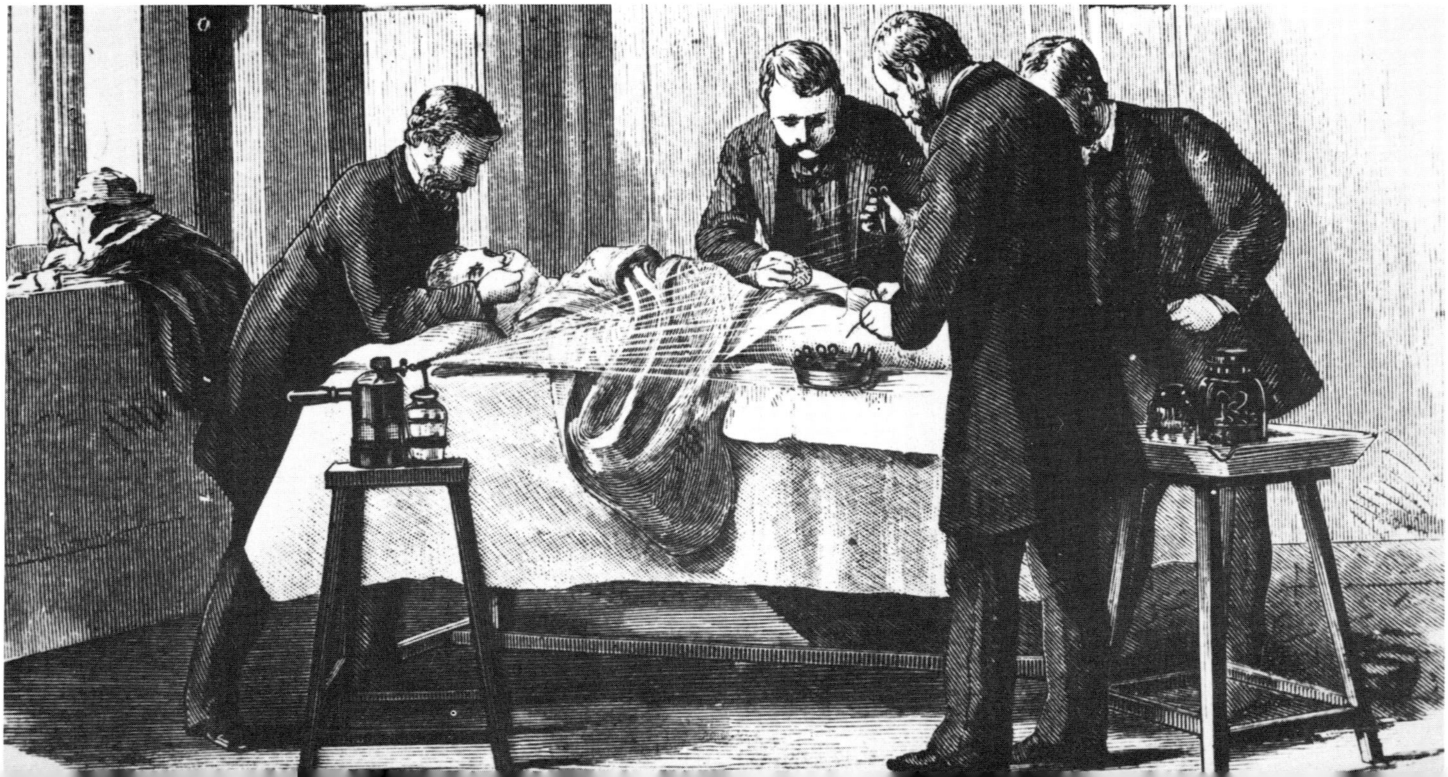

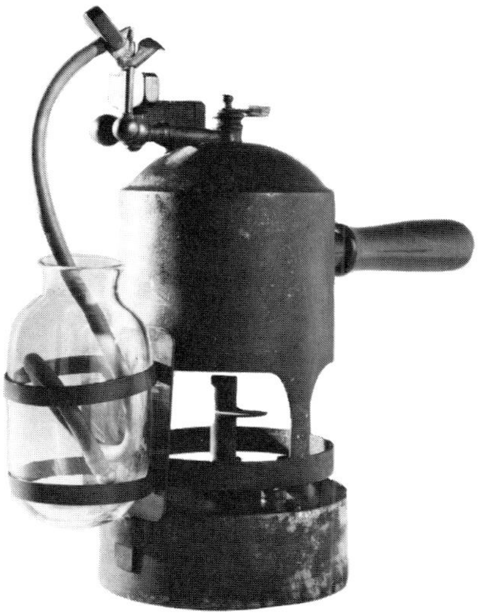

D A carbolic spray invented by Lister. The whole room would be sprayed with carbolic acid to prevent infection when operations were being carried out. The spray did work but the acid hurt the surgeon's eyes so Lister eventually stopped using it.

In 1877, therefore, when Lister moved from Glasgow to become Professor of Surgery at Kings College Hospital in London, many surgeons refused to put his ideas into practice. Nurses and surgeons complained that it took too long to keep washing everything. In any case, they refused to believe that infection was spread by dirty operating theatres and tools. People who have new ideas are often regarded as odd. A famous London surgeon at the time could often get a laugh by saying to his students, 'Shut the door quickly or one of Mr Lister's microbes may come in.'

F An operating theatre today

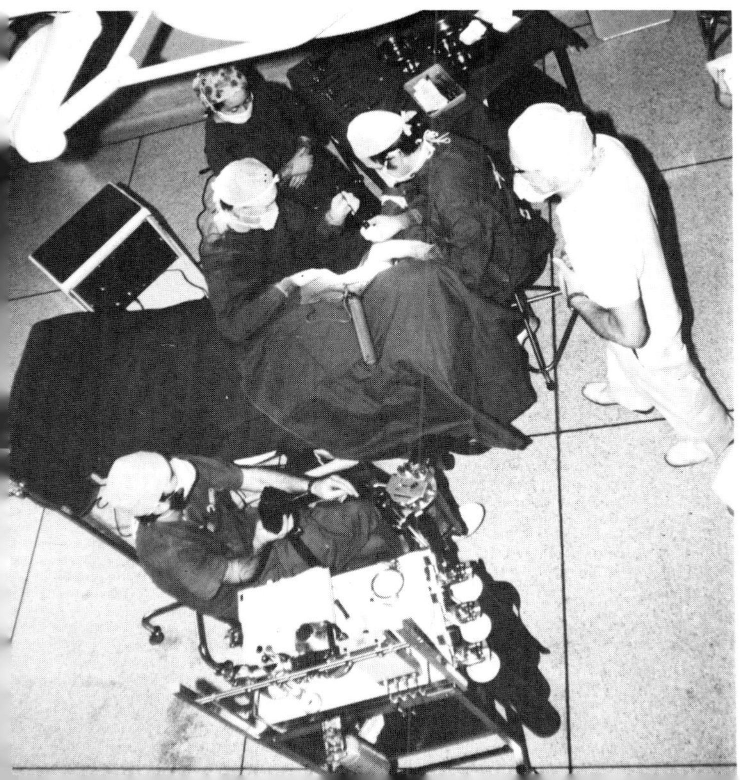

But Lister's ideas were accepted in the end. Today hospitals are careful that everything is kept very clean. If you visited a hospital today you would be certain to see germ-free or *sterile* instruments, swabs, gauze bandages and rubber gloves, and uniformed surgeons. Lister did not bring about all these improvements but he certainly paved the way for them.

???????????????????

1 Match the tails with the heads of these statements.

HEADS

Before Lister, many patients died because . . .

Most doctors at the time of Lister thought that . . .

Lister helped to prevent blood poisoning by insisting that . . .

Lister's methods of cleanliness have become known as . . .

TAILS

a poisonous mist in the air caused disease.

hands, bandages and surgeons' clothes should be kept very clean.

antiseptic surgery.

bacteria infected wounds and caused blood poisoning.

2 Look at the evidence and text in chapter 22. Say whether the statements below are true or false and give examples to prove your case.

a Before Lister, patients had a good chance of recovering from an operation (look at **A** in particular).
b Lister never gave up (look at **B** in particular).
c People were willing to accept Lister's ideas (look at **E** in particular).

3 List three reasons why people might have been hostile towards Lister and his ideas. Why might their views change in time?

4 Look at pictures **C** and **E.** Draw up a table like the one below

	In Lister's Time	Today
Number of helpers		
Clothes being worn		
Equipment		
Surgeons' hands		
Surgeons' mouths		

23 Obstetrics and Gynaecology

Do you know anyone who has had or is having a baby? Do you think they would have liked to have their baby during any of the periods mentioned in **A**? If not, why not?

A	
Period	**Attitudes to childbirth methods**
Ancient Egypt and Greece	Men never attended the confinement (the time when women are actually giving birth) because it was believed to be improper.
Roman Empire	The Romans made some progress. Seranus (AD 98-138) wrote a book on gynaecology (the science of women's diseases and pregnancy) with some sound advice about abortion and contraception. It was still, however, not easy or safe to give birth.
Muslim Empire	Albicasis, the great Muslim surgeon (see chapter 11), offered advice to midwives during confinement by standing behind a curtain so that he would not actually be able to see what was happening. He advised what is known today as 'watcher's position', where the woman lies with her hips at the edge of a table and lets her legs dangle. Albicasis also invented some forceps and other obstetrical instruments that were used throughout the Middle Ages.
Middle Ages in Europe	Trotula, a woman doctor at the medical school at Salerno, wrote a book on gynaecology. Midwives still did not want men near a woman during a confinement.
The Renaissance	In 1513 a book, *Rosegarden of pregnant women and midwives,* by Eucharius Roesslin contains no new ideas but served as the standard textbook on obstetrics (childbirth) for 200 years. It is unlikely that the author ever attended a childbirth. **B** shows one strange idea about childbirth at this time.

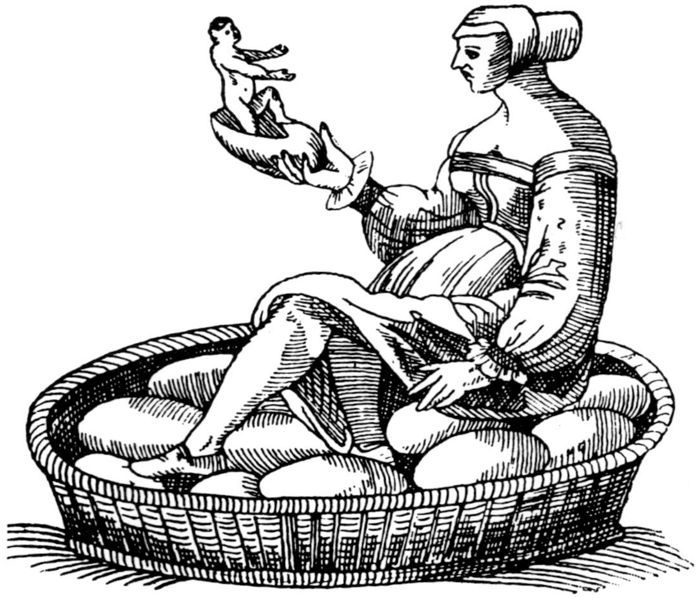

B Hatching children from eggs: one strange misunderstanding of childbirth.

According to **A** how much progress in obstetrics and gynaecology had been made by the end of the Renaissance? **C** shows a typical childbirth scene in about 1540 (during the Renaissance). Men are let into the

C A childbirth scene in 1540

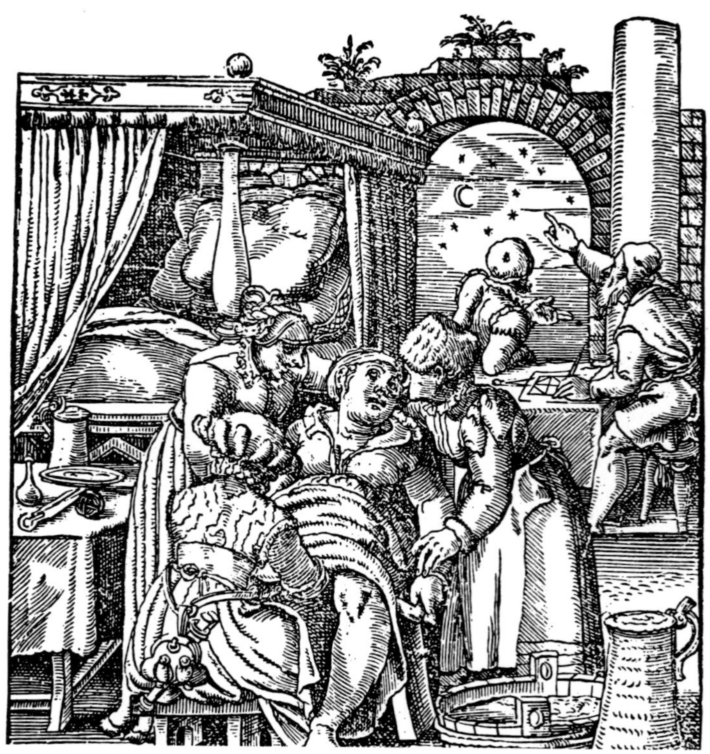

chamber but they stand a discreet distance away, and do not watch or take part in the delivery. They consult the stars to see what the child's future will be. The mother squats on a 'birth stool' and is helped by midwives.

It was through the determined efforts of Dr William Smellie (1697-1763) that trained doctors began to learn about childbirth and that midwives were properly trained. **D** describes what Smellie did:

❛ *He came to London in 1739. Although he was a complete stranger he began to give courses for midwives in his own home. Smellie's classes were successful. For his practice, this daring 'male midwife' had to rely at first on the poor. In their homes Smellie always gave his best. In one difficult labour case he reported, 'I sweated so much I was obliged to throw off my waistcoat and wig and put on my nightgown with a thin napkin over my head.'* ❜ (**D**)

A Pictorial History of Medicine *by O. Bettmann*

Smellie faced great opposition from midwives and doctors but he fought hard to convince people that the art of delivering a baby needed improving. In 1753 he wrote his *Treatise on Midwifery*. It was this book that gradually improved the standards of midwifery in Britain.

Ignatz Semmelweis was a Hungarian doctor of the 1840s who made childbirth more hygienic and safe. **E** describes how he did this:

❛ *In 1844, when he came to the maternity department of the Vienna General Hospital, the mortality (death) figures were shocking. In Ward one, attended by medical students, the death-rate was over 10 per cent. But in Ward eleven, which was set aside for the training of midwives, the rate was only 3 per cent. Semmelweis concluded that students coming to the ward from the dissecting room transmitted cadaveric* (from corpses) *matter into the system of pregnant women. The nurses in Ward eleven handled no autopsies, and this obviously accounted for the more favourable conditions there.*

Semmelweis took exceedingly simple measures to stop the deathmarch in Ward one. In May 1847, he asked his students to wash their hands in chlorinated lime water, and to scrub their fingernails with a handbrush before entering the ward. The death-rate in this ward then stood at 12.4 per cent. Within two months it fell to 1.27 per cent. ❜ (**E**)

A Pictorial History of Medicine *by O. Bettmann*

Like Lister, he found his colleagues opposed his ideas. They refused to believe that germs could be carried on the hands and cause death during pregnancies.

In America, Oliver Wendell Holmes came to a similar conclusion to Semmelweis's and was more successful in bringing his methods to obstetrics (childbirth). It is because of the efforts of men like Smellie, Semmelweis and Holmes that childbirth is now so much safer (**F**).

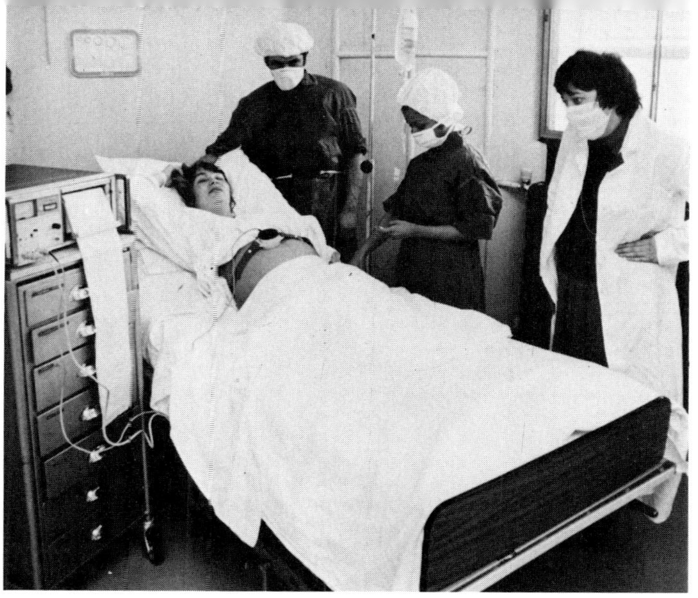

F A mother having a baby today has expert help from nurses, midwives and doctors, and babies are delivered in warm, sterile conditions.

??????????????????

1 Explain the meaning of each of the following: obstetrics, gynaecology, midwife, confinement.

2 Look at **C** and **F** and complete a chart like the one below:

	Childbirth in 1540	Childbirth today
Number of women in the room		
Number of men in the room		
Number of men helping with the delivery		
Aids being used		
Anaesthetic available?		
Dangers		

3 Five books are mentioned in Chapter 23. Give the title (if known) and author of each and say what influence (if any) each book had. Which are primary and which secondary sources?

4 Who were **a** William Smellie and **b** Ignatz Semmelweis? Describe the effect each man had on the development of obstetrics and gynaecology.

24 Florence Nightingale

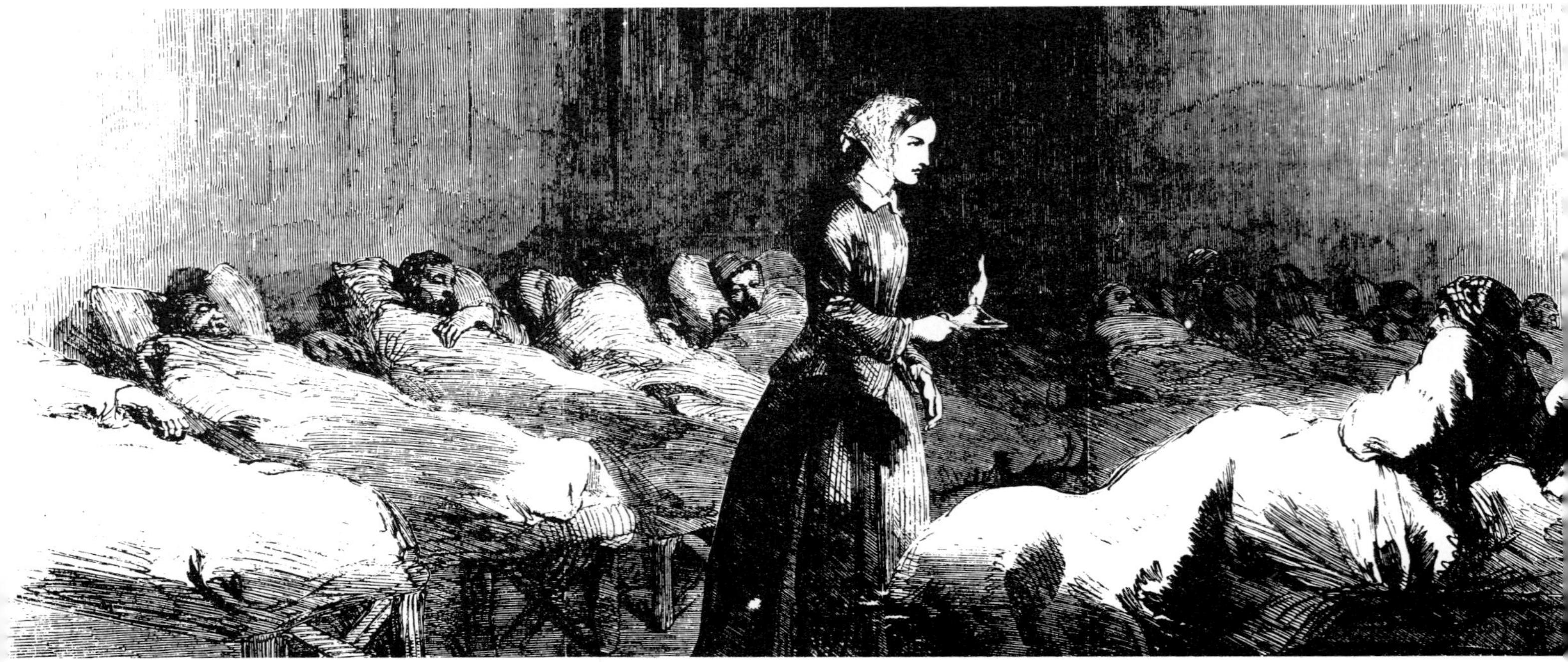

A Florence Nightingale inspects injured troops at night in the military hospital in Scutari during the Crimean War (1853-56).

You might have seen pictures like **A** before on the backs of ten pound notes. The picture shows Florence Nightingale (1820-1910) nursing troops at night. The scene is in a military hospital in Scutari in the Crimea during the Crimean war of 1853-56. **B** shows some of the changes in standards of nursing that Florence Nightingale helped bring about.

B Nurses before and after Florence Nightingale

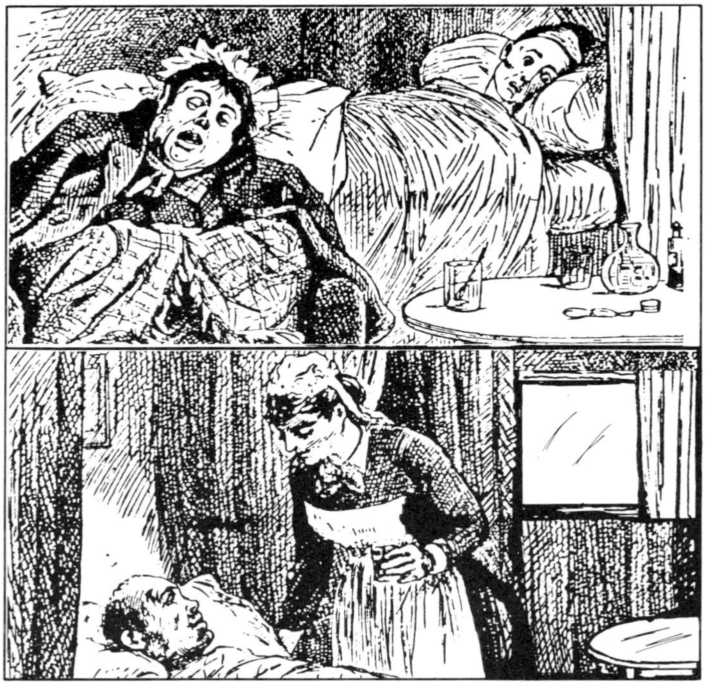

You will have read in chapter 7 that the Romans had superb military hospitals, and in chapter 11 about the hospitals in the Arab Empire. But, before Florence Nightingale, standards of nursing were very poor. During the Middle Ages the monasteries were almost the only places in Europe where hospitals could be found. In the sixteenth century, Henry VIII destroyed nearly all monasteries in England and from then on, nuns did most of the nursing that was available. This is why nurses today are called sisters. The most common complaints (before the 1850s) about nurses who were not nuns were that they were dirty or drunk. Nursing in 1850 was not a job that many respectable ladies would choose.

Florence Nightingale, however, was a respectable young lady from a wealthy family. She did more than anyone else at the time to improve standards of nursing and make them what they are today. On 9 October 1854 she read the following report in *The Times* about conditions faced by injured soldiers fighting in the Crimea:

❛ *No sufficient preparations have been made for the care of the wounded. Not only are there not sufficient surgeons, but there is not even linen to make bandages for the wounded. Men are kept in some cases for a week without a medical man coming near their wounds.* ❜ (**C**)

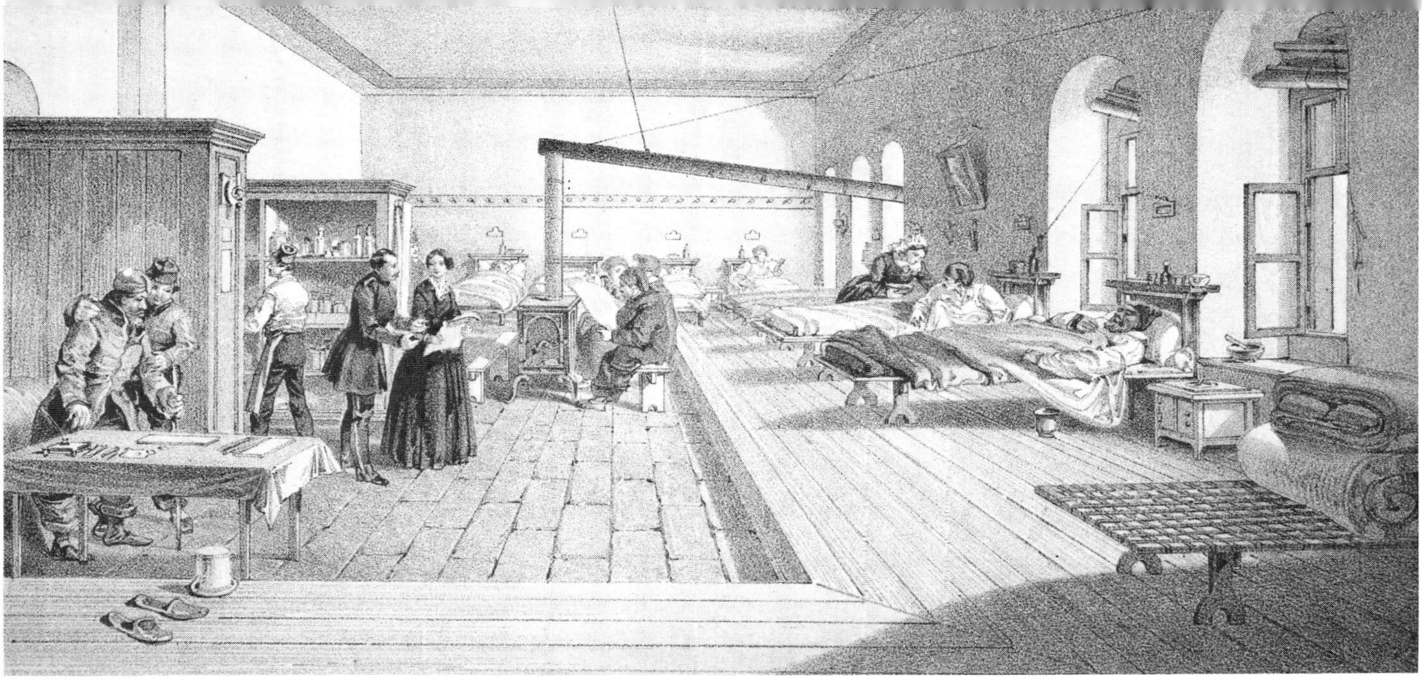

E The ward at Scutari after Florence Nightingale had made her improvements.

Florence (with the help of money from the government) gathered a group of 38 nurses together. She took them across Europe to Scutari in the Crimea (Russia) to help out. When they arrived they saw that conditions were even worse than *The Times* had suggested. Sarah Terrot, one of her nurses, wrote:

❛ *The scene baffles description. Horror upon horror crowds upon my mind . . . the misery of the dying was also aggravated by the vermin . . . Night is especially trying . . . At this period there were no night nurses, but Miss Nightingale, lamp in hand, each night traversed alone the four miles of beds.* ❜ **(D)**

Many army medical doctors resented the women nurses being there. At first, they were not allowed to do anything except prepare dressings and cook food. But when the casualties increased the nurses were slowly allowed to help out. Florence seized the opportunity. She insisted that the floors of the hospital were scrubbed and that the linen was always kept clean. She made sure all the nurses had tidy uniforms, that there was plenty of space between the beds, medicine in the cupboards and fresh air through open windows. When she first arrived 42 out of every 100 patients admitted to the hospital died. Within two years she had reduced the death rate to 2 in every 100.

When she returned to England in 1856 she was famous because she had proved that proper nursing could save lives. A public fund was set up and more than £50,000 was raised for her to set up the Nightingale School of Nursing in 1860 in a wing of St Thomas's hospital in London. Many doctors opposed this because they thought it was a criticism of their own work and that nurses were not really needed. Very soon, however, the school helped to establish nursing as a respectable profession.

Training at the school was strict: the nurses were only allowed to go out in pairs; they had to live in at the hospital and they had to keep a diary that was inspected every month. Many similar schools were opened and by 1901 there were 68000 trained nurses in Britain. whereas in 1850 there had been none. In 1919 the General Nursing Council was set up and today the SRN (State Registered Nurse) is considered vital in any hospital. Florence Nightingale began all this.

??????????????????

1 Use **A** as well as information in the text to describe what nursing was like up to the time of Florence Nightingale. Suggest some reasons why it was so bad.

2 What are the main differences in nursing shown in the two pictures in source **B**? Mention: attentiveness, cleanliness, soberness, uniform and any other points.

3 Describe what conditions were like at Scutari before Florence Nightingale went there.

4 Name five improvements that Florence Nightingale made that are shown in **E**. Say how each of these improvements would have helped to save lives.

5 *'Nursing in 1850 was not a job that many respectable young ladies would choose.'* Why not? Describe how Florence Nightingale changed this.

25 Public Health 1800-1900

By 1850 many important advances in medicine had been made. Yet, if you had been born in the early or middle part of the nineteenth century you could not expect to live beyond the age of forty. People who lived in industrial towns had more children than most people do today and two out of every ten babies died soon after birth. Epidemic diseases (diseases which spread very quickly) killed thousands of people every year. The table below shows deaths in Britain from cholera epidemics (cholera is a disease caused by germs in water):

A	
Year	**Deaths from cholera epidemics**
1833	22,000
1848-49	72,000
1853-54	20,000
1866	14,500

Some of the cures doctors suggested for cholera included opium, tobacco, strychnine, ice-cold baths and boiling hot baths. Other major diseases of the time that killed thousands of people each year included smallpox, measles and diphtheria. Tuberculosis killed between 50,000 and 60,000 a year.

B–**F** are all primary sources showing what living conditions were like in the larger towns during the nineteenth century. As more and more people moved into the towns after the Industrial Revolution (see chapter 19), there were greater demands for water and for sewage disposal. Many town councils did not seem to realize that something needed to be done to clean up the towns and improve living conditions.

B Slums on an island in the river Thames in the 1840s

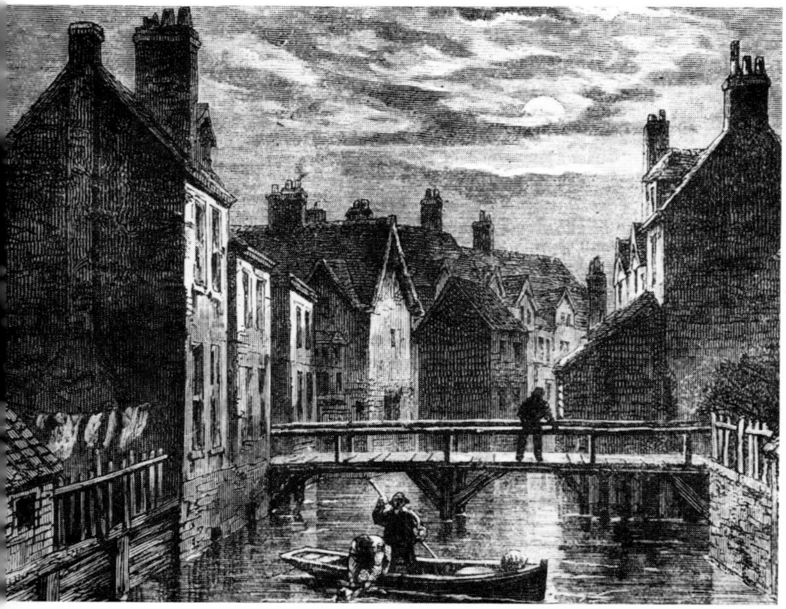

B shows what conditions were like in working-class districts. This district was surrounded by a foul ditch into which people tipped rubbish and sewage. The ditch was also the main water supply for the area. **C** is a description of a similar area in 1849 where two boys had died within a week of each other in a house in Rochester:

❛ *The evidence showed that the cellar, to the depth of at least six inches, is covered with all kinds of refuse, that the spout from the privy, that runs through the cellar, is broken and everything falls through to the cellar.* ❜ (**C**)

Many streets and houses were filthy. Sewers which ran down the middle of the streets were not wide enough to carry off the slops. Even when they were, the sewage flowed into the rivers. The rivers were the main source of drinking water. It is not surprising that cholera spread when people got their water from the pumps shown in **D.**

Two hundred people might share one toilet at the end of the street. Cellars like the one described in **C** might be inhabited by ten or more people. The houses of the middle class often looked cleaner than those of the working class but were in some cases just as likely to be breeding grounds for disease.

The smell of the sewage in the streets was terrible (**E**). **F** is a letter written by an MP in 1857:

❛ *Sir,*
Will you permit me to draw your attention to the pestilential state of the atmosphere at times in and about the new Houses of Parliament, owing to the evaporation of sewage matter in the Thames on hot sunny days? The stench arising from the river has on several occasions compelled me to leave the terrace and I am frequently obliged to close all the windows of my office to exclude if possible the noisome air, the subtle poison of which, however, penetrates everywhere, causing headache, nausea and loss of appetite. This state of things must be most injurious to the health of members of Parliament. ❜ (**F**)

At this time people knew little about how diseases spread. Leading doctors and surgeons knew that dirty conditions were linked to disease, but the general public and the authorities did little about it.

D This diagram, from a book by Dr J. Snow, shows deaths from cholera in a small area of London during a period of 11 days in 1854. A mark or bar is placed on the house where deaths from cholera took place. The deaths all centre on the pump in Broad Street.

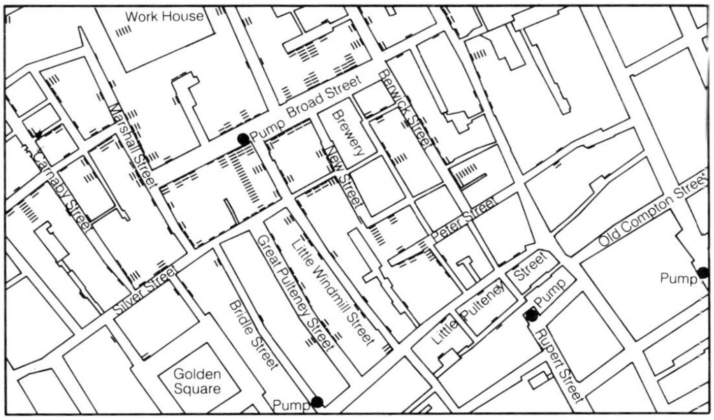

?????????????????

1 Imagine you are producing a report for the government on Public Health during the nineteenth century and you have been given the evidence in these pages. Present your report under the following headings (you may include drawings and diagrams in your report):

- **a** Description of streets
- **b** Description of working-class living conditions
- **c** Evidence of deaths from diseases
- **d** The problems of sewage disposal
- **e** The problems of water supply
- **f** Suggested action to be taken

2 a Which of the evidence **A–F** do you think tells us most about Public Health in the nineteenth century? What does it tell us?

b What do you think was the main reason for the deaths shown in **D**? Explain your answer.

3 Look back to chapter 7 and compare Public Health facilities in Roman times with those in nineteenth century Britain. You could do it in the form of a chart like this:

	Roman times	Nineteenth century
Water Streets Houses etc	Piped in aqueducts	Pumped out of river

E This cartoon of 1849 offers a way for people walking the streets to avoid the smell of the sewers, by sniffing the purer air further up.

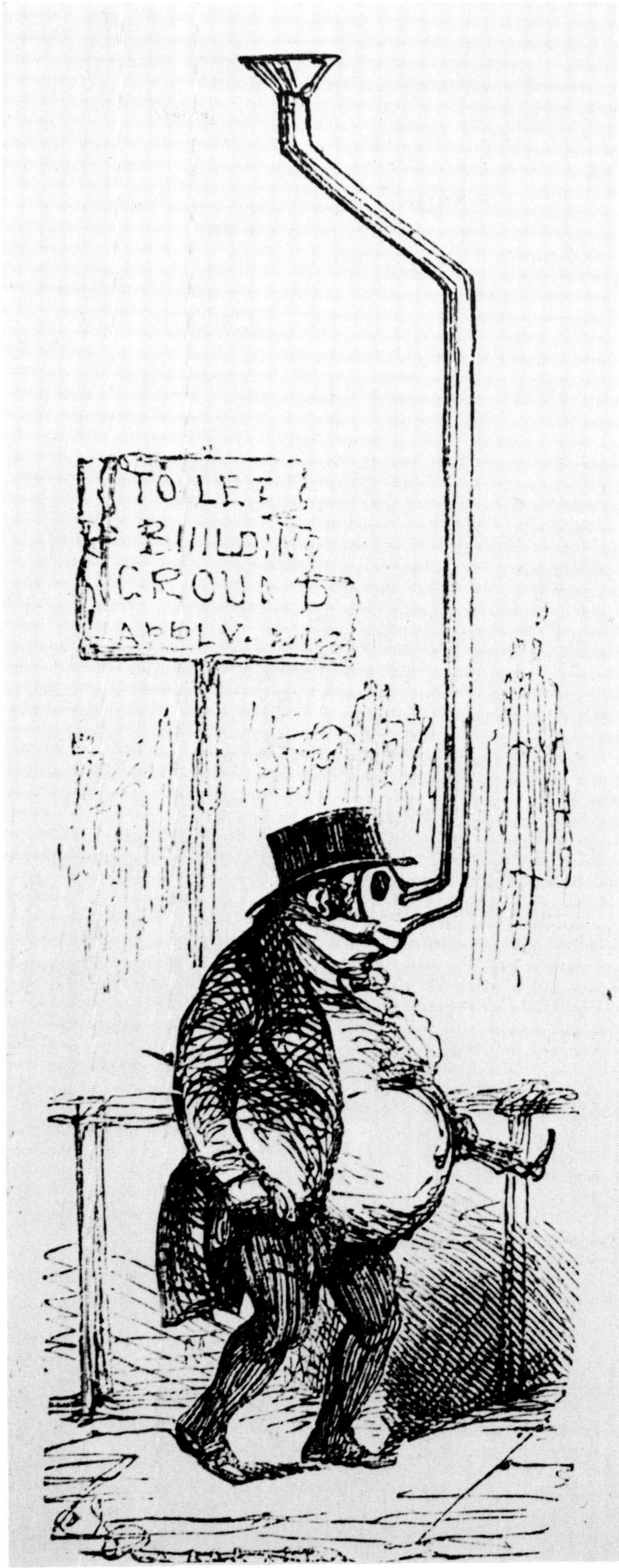

26 Public Health Reform

A	Acts affecting Public Health

1848 Public Health Act Any town could have a Public Health Board if it wanted one or if one tenth of the ratepayers demanded it. The Central Board of Health in London could force towns to have a Public Health Board only if the death rate in the town was as high as 23 in every 1000. The Boards had the power to set a rate for proper drainage and sewage disposal and for cleaning the streets.

By 1854 Chadwick and the Public Health Board had persuaded 182 towns to set up boards.

1854 Chadwick's Public Health Board was closed down.

1855 Board of Health set up again with John Simon at its head.

1864 Factory Act forced employers to guard against unhealthy conditions in factories, such as lack of ventilation.

1866 Sanitary Act Every town had to have Sanitary Inspectors with powers to order landlords to stop overcrowding and to remove health hazards from their properties.

1875 Public Health Act allowed Authorities to pull down slums. There had to be a Public Health Committee in every district and they had to provide water, get rid of sewage, inspect food and markets, clear away rubbish and put a stop to unhealthy conditions in work places. Towns had to have a Health Inspector and a Sanitary Officer.

Local and central government at the beginning of the nineteenth century believed in *laissez-faire*. Laissez-faire is French for 'leave alone' and this is what they thought the government should do: leave things alone and not enforce change.

A shows that slowly this attitude began to alter and that by 1875 the government was forcing the towns to improve their public health services such as sewage and lighting. These changes were largely the work of a small number of men who convinced the government that improving public health would save lives. A leader among them was Jeremy Bentham, who spread the idea that a government should pass an act only if it would be of use to the majority of the population. Edwin Chadwick, who believed in Bentham's ideas, became Secretary of a commission looking into the Poor Law in 1832. The main place where poor people could receive medical attention was in a workhouse (**B**). Chadwick was in charge of workhouses after 1834. He reported that the workhouses had to look after thousands of people every time there was an epidemic. He decided to find out why this was so and his investigations revealed the dirty and unhealthy conditions described in chapter 25.

His report on public health, published in 1842, contained figures like **C**:

Average age of death	**Manchester** (town)	**Rutland** (country)
Gentry and professional people	38	52
Tradesmen and farmers	20	41
Labourers	17	38

Chadwick believed that sewers and drains would solve all public health problems. He even backed the idea of emptying London's sewage into the Thames. The Thames was used as drinking water. **D** gives some extracts from his report of 1842:

❛ *. . . that the various forms of epidemic . . . are caused, or aggravated . . . chiefly among the labouring classes by atmospheric impurities produced by decomposing animal and vegetable substances, by damp and filth, and close and overcrowded dwellings . . . Where these circumstances are removed by drainage, proper cleansing, better ventilation . . . the frequency and intensity of such disease is reduced.* ❜ (**D**)

Some of Chadwick's ideas were taken into account in the Public Health Act 1848 (**A**), but its measures were not compulsory. He met a great deal of opposition when trying to set up Public Health Boards. Local businessmen only wanted to improve the wealthy districts, and water companies complained that they would lose profits. His opponents became nicknamed 'The Dirty Party'. They complained that his ideas meant too much government interference.

But Chadwick convinced many MPs that his ideas were right. John Simon (see **A**) continued Chadwick's work. Slowly the government began to change its attitude. Cholera epidemics (see chapter 25) convinced many MPs that something needed to be done. In 1875 the new Public Health Act forced towns to make the changes that were necessary and laid the foundations for the Public Health Service of today.

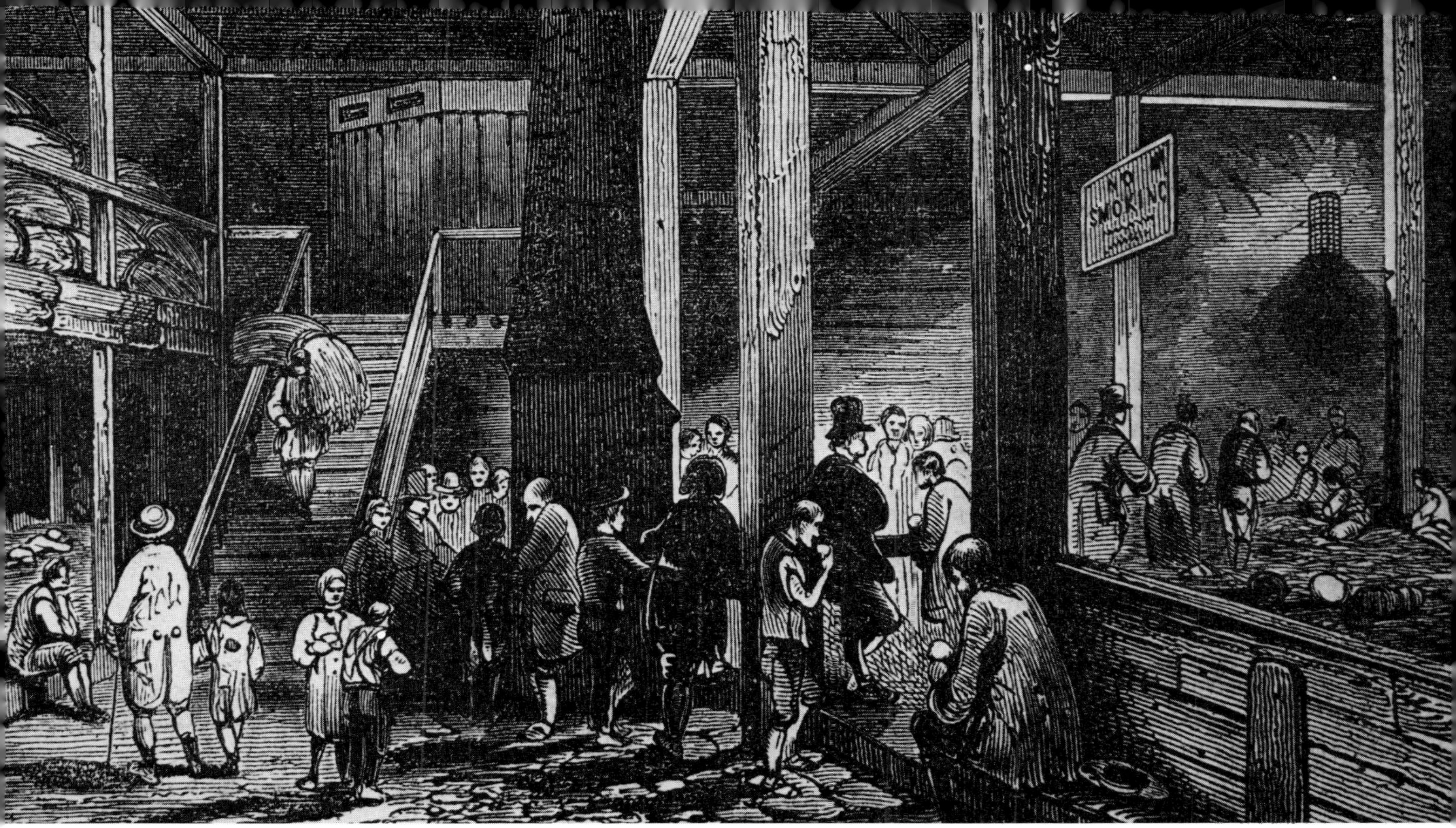

B The male ward in a workhouse. Poor people had to go to workhouses if they were ill, could not find work or support themselves. Patients were usually looked after by other unqualified inmates.

E A workman in a bleaching factory is overcome by inhaling fumes. Which of the acts in **A** would have helped to put a stop to this sort of problem?

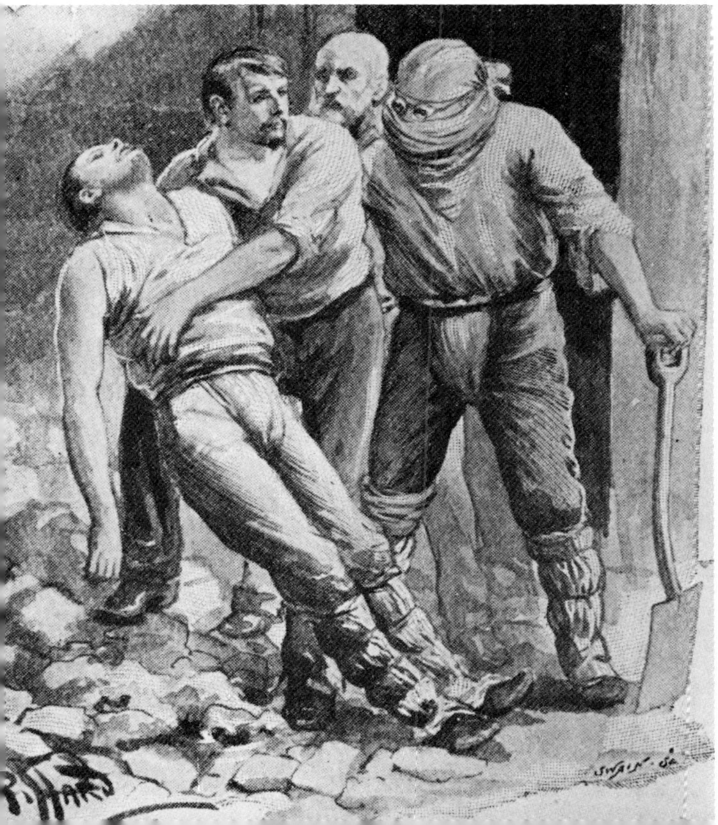

??????????????????

1 List the different ways of improving public health that are mentioned in **A**. Which one do you think would have had the most effect and why?

2 Comment on the standard of medical care poor people could get in the early nineteenth century (see **B**). Mention cleanliness, doctors, nurses, medicines, etc.
Compare this with the help poor people can get today.

3 Show the information in **C** as a graph and explain what it tells us about the difference between town life (in Manchester) and country life (in Rutland).

4 a What suggestions did Edwin Chadwick make about how to improve Public Health?
b What opposition did Chadwick meet and why was there so much?

5 *The Public Health Act of 1848 shows that a laissez-faire approach to government was being taken. The Public Health Act of 1875 shows that this attitude had changed.*
Explain how and why this change happened. Mention: what laissez-faire was, why governments began to change their minds (e.g., the work of Bentham, Chadwick and Simon); epidemics and why the 1875 act was not a laissez-faire act.

27 Mental Illness

A Care of the Mentally Ill	
Year/Period	**Main ideas or developments**
Prehistoric times	Trephining operation (see chapter 1) might have been carried out to release 'demons' from the head, although we have no proof of this.
Ancient Greece	Hippocrates treated the mentally ill with kindness and recommended vapour baths and exercise.
Middle Ages	**B** shows the screw-like device used during the Middle Ages to allow demons to escape from heads of people who were probably mentally ill. The Royal Bethlehem Hospital (Bedlam) was opened for mental patients in 1369 (see **C**).
Eighteenth century	Mental patients were regarded as criminals and often treated like the patient in **C**.
Nineteenth century	The nineteenth century saw the beginning of a slightly more humane attitude to mental patients but progress was slow.
1793	Philippe Pinel ordered that all the mental patients in the Bicentre Hospital in Paris should be released from their chains.
1795	William Tuke opened the Retreat Mental Hospital in York. Patients were given as much freedom as possible to move around. The methods of Pinel and Tuke were also carried out by Jean Equinol (1772-1840) in France, John Conolly (1794-1860) in England, and Thomas Kirkbride (1809-93) and Dorothea Lynd-Dix (1802-1887) in America.
1863	Lord Shaftesbury opened Broadmoor prison in England where criminals and mentally ill criminals were separated for the first time in English prisons.

Have you ever heard anyone say that they are 'worried sick' about something? Maybe when you get excited about something or nervous, you get a funny feeling in your stomach or you don't feel like eating. Doctors now believe that the way you feel or think can actually affect your health. In other words, your mind can control your body. This is a fairly recent discovery, as **A** shows:

A shows how attitudes towards the treatment of the mentally ill changed very slowly. Why do you think this was so? **C** describes conditions in Bedlam as late as 1895.

B Trephining was still carried out in the Middle Ages but by this time a screw-like device was used. The hole allowed demons to escape from the brain.

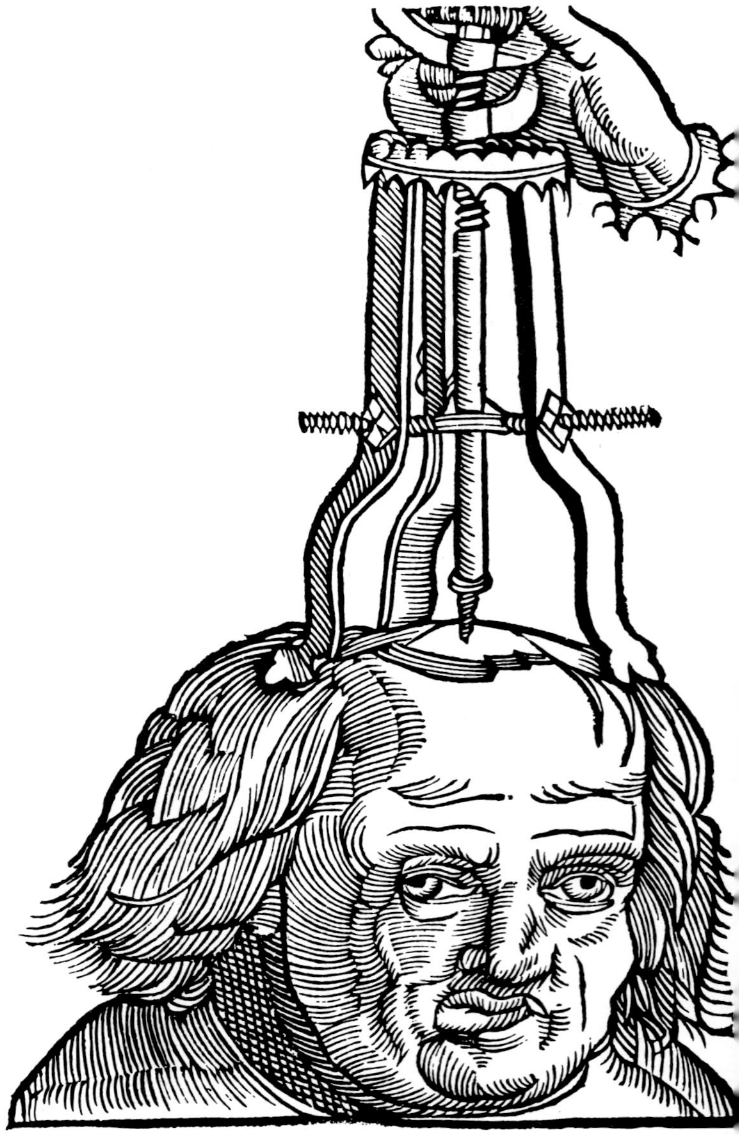

❛ *One of the side rooms contained about ten patients, each chained by one arm or leg to the wall, the chain allowed them merely to stand up by the bench or form fixed to the wall, or to sit down on it.*

One man named William Norris . . . had been kept for nine years fastened to the wall with chains and an iron bar which prevented him moving more than twelve inches away from it. ❜ (**C**)

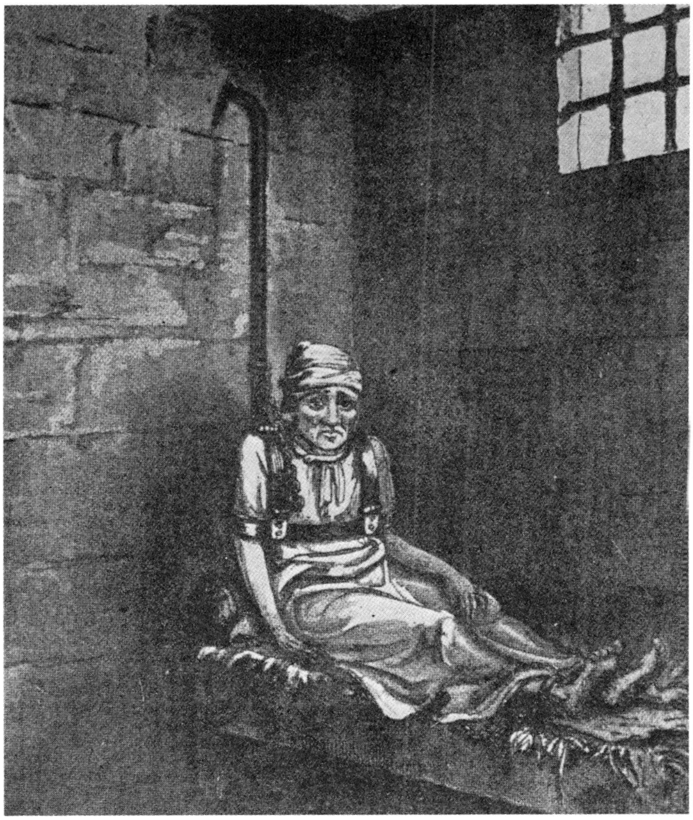

D A patient in 'Bedlam' (a mental hospital) in the early nineteenth century, is restrained with manacles and chained to the wall.

Even the new 'freer' methods favoured by Pinel and Tuke might still seem cruel to us today, as **E** shows. Chains and beatings might have gone but the strait jacket took their place.

❛ *Special basket contraptions were invented . . . in which the patient was encased from his neck to his thighs; this bizarre means kept his arms attached to his sides but did not prevent him from walking around. Wooden boxes were also devised for inmates who threatened suicide. They were five and a half feet long, two feet wide and eighteen inches deep and the insides were padded with straw. The madman was placed inside this contraption and was kept in place by means of the lid which was shut upon him in such a way that only his head, which he was unable to withdraw into the box, continued to stick out.* ❜ (**E**)

The major advances in the treatment of the mentally ill have taken place during the twentieth century with the use of drugs to calm and even cure some mental patients. **F** and **G** show other methods which help both doctor and patient understand their mental problems; they are based on the work of Sigmund Freud (1856-1939).

❛ *As a rule it is necessary to hypnotize the patient and to arouse his memories of the time at which the symptom made its first appearance. The symptoms we have been able to trace back (and cure by this method) include hysterical attacks, epileptic fits, chronic vomiting and anorexia (a desire not to eat).* ❜ (**F**)

From Preliminary Connection *in* Joint Studies in Hysteria
by Brewer and Freud

❛ *The true meaning of the dream is always intelligible; it has its starting point in experiences of the previous day, and proves to be a fulfilment of unsatisfied wishes. You will also learn with astonishment from the analysis of dreams what a great part is played in human developments by impressions and experiences of early childhood.* ❜ (**G**)

From Five letters on Psycho-analysis
by Freud

?????????????????

1 Complete a chart like the one below. Include information about the eight people mentioned in the text.

Pioneers of new attitudes to mental illness		
Name	**Country**	**What they did for the mentally ill**
Philippe Pinel 1745-1826	France	Released them from their chains
William Tuke 1732-1822		

2 It is the nineteenth century. Imagine that you have been put into a mental hospital by mistake. Use **D** and **E** to help you write some extracts in a diary over a period of about four years, showing the treatment you receive. Your warders think you are violent and might commit suicide.

3 Write a description of the changing methods of treating mental illness from prehistoric times to the present day.

4 Describe the ways in which mental illness is treated today. Mention: drugs, and psycho-analysis. Say how each method differs from the next and which you believe is the best.

28 The Growth of Hospitals

A	Major hospitals in Britain 1700-1900
1719	Westminster hospital founded
1725	Guy's hospital in London founded
1733	St George hospital in London founded
1739	Foundling hospital in Bloomsbury (London) founded by Thomas Coram
1740	The London hospital founded
1745	Middlesex hospital founded
1795	The Retreat mental hospital in York founded by William Tuke.
1814	London chest hospital opened
1828	Royal 'Free' hospital founded by William Marsden
1851	Royal (Marsden) cancer hospital opened
1852	Children's hospital opened in Great Ormond Street, London

There have been hospitals from early times. The Egyptians had healing centres, the Greeks had Asclepaeia and the Romans had advanced military hospitals. During the Middle Ages in Europe, the monasteries had hospital wings, and in the Arab Empire there were superb hospitals like the one at Baghdad (see chapter 11). In France, the famous Hôtel-Dieu hospital was founded as early as AD 660, but Britain lagged behind. The few hospitals that existed were under the control of the church.

Hospitals began to increase in number (**A**) as towns grew in size because of the Industrial Revolution. Yet in 1800 there were only 3000 patients in hospitals in England and Wales and by 1851 this figure had only risen to 7619. You have seen how dangerous it was to have an operation before the use of anaesthetics or antiseptics, so it is not surprising that people were afraid to go into hospital.

In the early nineteenth century, people had to pay to go into a hospital even though the conditions were so bad. Poor people went to workhouses (see chapter 26) or 'Charity' hospitals where their local parish or church might pay the bill for them. The surgeons in these wards were well paid, but **B** shows what the conditions were like.

❛ *Filth was universal. The patients wore the same shirts for seven weeks; bedding was only changed and washed once a month; food was at starvation level; spirits (alcohol) entered into the infirmary freely.* ❜ (**B**)

Some doctors in country areas set up small cottage hospitals for patients who could pay. Slowly the Poor Law (workhouse) hospitals began to copy the high standards set by these cottage hospitals. By the 1890s many charity hospitals had become teaching hospitals (see **C**). More trained doctors and surgeons were needed because of the increasing population (see chapter 19). As better training became available (see chapter 29) and conditions improved, people began to trust hospitals a little more. Some of the rules in these new hospitals might seem strange to us today (see **D**).

C An operation in 1865. Trainee doctors watch the operation from the gallery in order to learn.

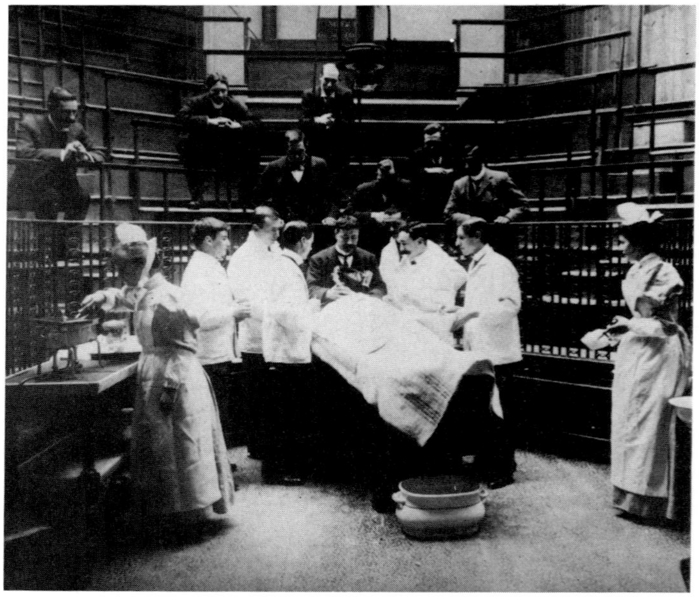

D	Rules of Guy's Hospital in the Nineteenth Century

1 Patients must address themselves morning and evening to God by prayer.
2 On Sunday evening between 6 and 8 some sober person should read a chapter from the Old Testament and a chapter from the New Testament.
3 Any person using lewd language three times shall be dismissed.
4 If any patient be found strolling about the streets or frequenting Public Houses they forfeit their next day's diet.
5 If any patient is found smoking in bed they are to be discharged.

29 Medical Education

A is about the training of doctors from 1518-1956. It is a secondary source. What does it tell us about the growth of medical education?

❛ *Though St Bartholomew's hospital began its medical school in 1662 and the Edinburgh medical school dates from 1736, medical training in the eighteenth century was mainly in the hands of doctors and surgeons . . . Westminster medical school dates from 1834 and St Mary's from 1854 . . . The College of Physicians founded by Linacre in 1518 still survived. The Society of Apothecaries founded in 1617 could, after 1815 examine and license candidates as General Practitioners. In 1800 the Royal College of Surgeons was established.*

The first woman medical graduate received her degree at New York in 1849. She was Elizabeth Blackwell . . . In Britain, Elizabeth Garrett was the first woman to qualify as a doctor when, in 1865 she obtained the licence of the Society of Apothecaries.

On her (Florence Nightingale's) *return* (from the Crimean War of 1854-56.) *The Nightingale school was founded at St Thomas's Hospital . . . The General Nursing Council was set up in 1919 to register nurses . . . In 1863 there were only 110 paid nurses in the whole of London; now there are about 60,000.* ❜ (**A**)

From The Story of Medicine *by D.W. Sylvester 1979*

Pictures like **B** (a medieval drawing) show us how doctors often got their training up to the nineteenth century. They watched other doctors or learned what they could by observing and listening. Even in the late nineteenth century people who were ill often consulted untrained 'medics'. Barber-surgeons (see chapter 20) could perform simple operations. Apothecaries would see a patient and describe their condition to a physician who could prescribe a cure that the apothecary would make up. There were unlicensed doctors who visited the poor.

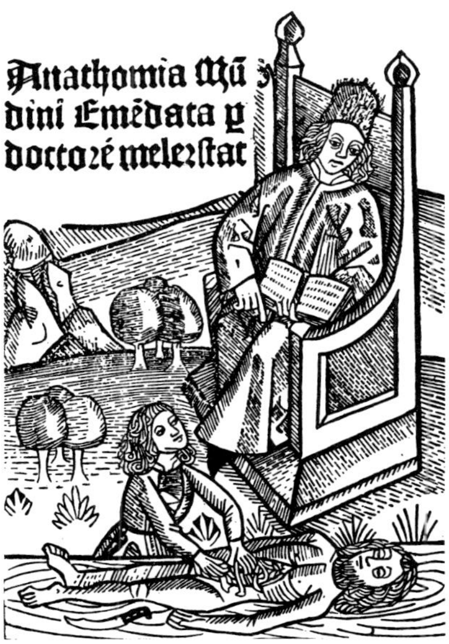

B Title page of a fifteenth-century anatomy book showing a student of anatomy following a doctor's instructions.

C shows the training that students do today before they can become doctors:

C **Curriculum**
1 *Basic medical science course* Two years training as a biological scientist. 2 *The special medical science course* One year study of one of the following options: Biochemistry, human morphology, microbiology, pathology, physiology, pharmacology. 3 *Clinical practice* Two years work as students on hospital wards or in laboratories etc.
From *Prospectus* for University of Nottingham's Medical School 1980-1981

As more hospitals were needed because of the increasing population more hospitals began to train people as doctors. Sometimes government action helped, for example, when the National Health Service was set up in 1948 (see chapter 34).

??????????????????

1 Say why hospitals were unpopular in 1800 but more popular in 1900. Mention: conditions, Lister, Nightingale, cottage hospitals, trained doctors.

2 Imagine you are one of the students in the gallery in **C.** Describe in detail the operation you are watching and say how hospitals are so much better now (i.e., in 1895) than when you were born (1850).

3 Write down the following dates from **A** and put by the side what happened in each year:
1518, 1617, 1662, 1736, 1815, 1834, 1849, 1854, 1856, 1863, 1865, 1919,
Now look at your list. What does it tell us about the development of medical education in Britain?

4 Find out the meaning of the words under the heading 'Curriculum' in **C.** Write an imaginary diary of some of the things you might see as a medical student at the University of Nottingham Medical School.

30 Koch, Ehrlich and Bacteriology

❛ . . . *the forehead covered with drops of sweat, the cheeks painted a livid crimson, the eyes sunk, the palms of the hands dry and painfully hot to the touch; the breath offensive, quick and laborious; and the cough so incessant as scarce to allow the wretched sufferer time to tell his complaints.* ❜ (**A**)

The novelist Charles Dickens wrote **A** to describe the disease tuberculosis (TB). In 1906 Albert Calnette and Camille Guerin discovered a vaccine against the TB germ – it became known as the BCG vaccine (Bacille Calnette-Guerin). Vaccines are made from the germs which cause the disease. Once a person has been vaccinated, the body builds up an immunity against these germs and will not catch the disease.

B Decline in annual death rate from diphtheria (above) and TB (below) in England and Wales

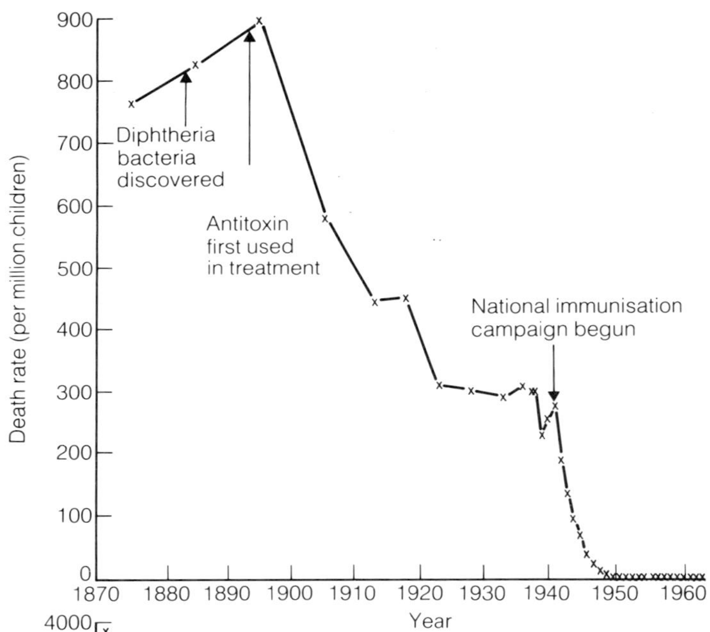

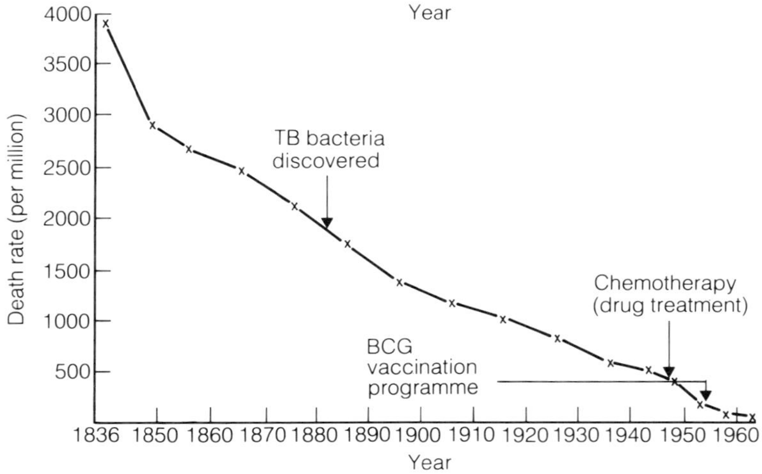

Anti-toxins also help fight disease. In 1890 Emil Behring discovered that blood serum from an animal which had recovered from diphtheria contained a substance which destroyed the poison (toxin) made by the diphtheria germ. He called this substance an anti-toxin. When injected into a diphtheria patient it helped cure the disease (see **B**).

They could not have made their discoveries if it had not been for the work of Robert Koch (1843-1910):

C	**Main achievements of Robert Koch**
1	Isolated the germs that cause anthrax.
2	1862 isolated TB germ.
3	1863 isolated cholera germ.
4	1880 isolated septicaemia (blood poisoning) germ.
5	He did not actually discover the cures for the diseases but by isolating the germs he made it easier for others to study them.

A modern historian described how Koch discovered the anthrax bacillus (germ):

❛ *Koch became a self-made bacteriologist after a year's work as district physician in Wollstein, Silesia. His laboratory experience was limited and his equipment simple, except perhaps for the microscope which Frau Koch had given him on his thirtieth birthday in 1873. In a corner of his office he set out to examine the blood of animals which had died in a local epidemic of anthrax. First, he tracked down its causative bacillus; then he succeeded in breeding it in a 'pure culture'. From this culture he could infect other animals at will. This closed the circle of evidence and proved that anthrax was caused by a specific microbe.* ❜ (**D**)

From A Pictorial History of Medicine *by Otto Bettmann*

Koch was a very patient man. After hundreds of experiments he discovered that if you took blood from an animal that had anthrax and injected it into a healthy animal then the healthy animal caught the disease. If he took blood from the second animal and injected it into a third, then the third animal also got the disease, but more quickly. The more times he did this, the stronger the anthrax bacteria became until eventually the anthrax microbes killed all the other germs in the blood. He was then able to isolate the anthrax microbe and grow a pure version of it on a glass plate. This made it much easier to study the germ.

Koch's work in isolating germs made it possible to study them carefully and therefore to find out exactly what caused the disease. This made it easier to find a cure, although Koch himself did not discover the cures for the diseases he studied (see **E**). The writer of **D** praised Koch by saying: 'If Pasteur had made bacteriology a science, Koch made it an exact one.' What do you think he meant by this? Do you agree?

Paul Ehrlich joined Koch's research team at the Institute for Infectious Diseases in Berlin in 1890. Koch had discovered that in some cases dyes could stain certain bacteria and make them easier to see. He had not been able to get very far, though, with this research. Ehrlich was fascinated by dyes and he tried out hundreds of them to see which bacteria they would seek out. This research led him to work out that the bloodstream has antibodies that kill particular germs. He called them 'magic bullets' because they sought out the germs they wanted to kill without harming others the body needs.

Ehrlich realised that he could use dyes to carry drugs to certain tissues only without them harming the other tissues on the way. His team's most startling discovery using this method was *Salvarsan 606* which killed many bacteria at the same time, including the one that caused syphilis. **F** describes how Ehrlich learnt of the discovery:

❛ *Having made his first experiments, Dr Hata came to show Ehrlich his records and said with his usual polite bows, 'Only first trials . . . only preliminary general view. Believe 606 very efficacious . . .'*

Ehrlich looked at the records and said, astonished, 'No, surely not? It was all minutely tested by Dr R and he found nothing, nothing . . . More than a year ago we laid aside 606 as being ineffective, worthless. You are sure you are not mistaken, Dr Hata?'

Hata pointed to the records of the experiments and said, shrugging his shoulders, 'I found that, Herr Geheimrat (director).' *'Then it must be repeated, dear Hata, repeated,' said Ehrlich.*

. . . One morning he came quickly into his laboratory, followed by Dr Hata. 'Well, my dear Hata, what have you found out now?' asked Ehrlich, coming nearer. With repeated nods of the head, Hata replied, 'Always 606 best.' 'Incredible,' said Ehrlich. 'What an incapable good-for-nothing!' he exclaimed, his big eyes looking at Dr Hata over the tops of his spectacles. Hata looked scared and stretched out his arms as if in defence. Ehrlich put his hand on Hata's shoulder, soothingly, and shook his head. 'Oh, not you,' he said, 'not you. No, the other fellow before you.'

Then Dr Hata beamed with delight and grinning broadly he repeated, 'The stupid good-for-nothing!' ❜ **(F)**

From Paul Ehrlich *by Martha Marquandt*

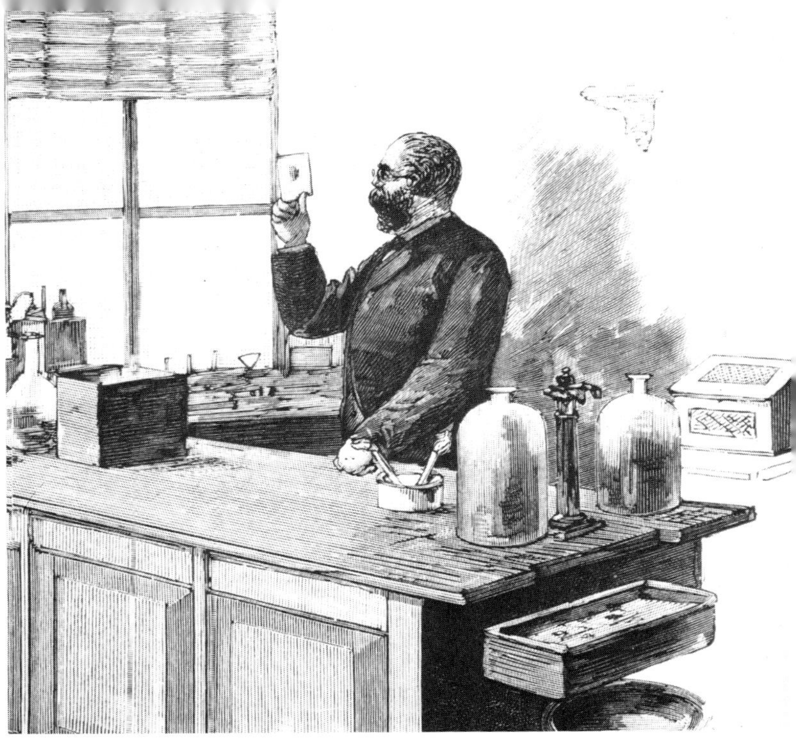

E Robert Koch at work in his laboratory

??????????????????

1 What disease is described in **A**? Who eventually discovered a cure for the disease?

2 Find evidence from the chapter that shows that Robert Koch was **a** patient, **b** methodical and **c** 'went one step further than Pasteur'.

3 What were the 'magic bullets', as Ehrlich called them? What discoveries concerning the use of dyes did these magic bullets lead to?

4 Look at **B:**
- **a** Describe how a cure for diphtheria was found.
- **b** What was the national immunisation campaign in the 1940s?
- **c** Name two things which accelerated (speeded up) the fall in the numbers of people dying from tuberculosis.

5 What does **F** tell us about the discovery of Salvarsan 606? Who do you think should take the credit for the discovery?

6 *The work of bacteriologists had more effect on saving peoples' lives than any other medical developments of the nineteenth century.*
What do you think? In your answer you should mention: the work of people such as Pasteur, Koch and Ehrlich, and you should decide whether their work had a greater effect than that of people such as Chadwick, Simpson, Lister, Nightingale, etc.

31 The Conquest of Infectious Disease

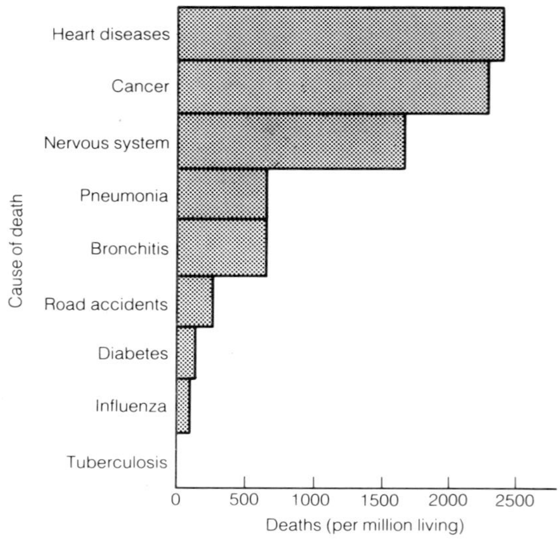

A The main causes of death in Britain between 1956 and 1966.

A shows that infectious disease is no longer a major cause of death in Britain. Chapter 30 looks at the discovery of cures for such diseases as tuberculosis and diphtheria. Discovering a cure or way of preventing the disease is only the first step, though, in eradicating (getting rid of) a disease altogether. This last has resulted from people's patient hard work and the cooperation of different countries.

Malaria is a good example. For thousands of years before 1900, malaria had been a killer disease. Today, it is quite rare for anyone to die of the disease. **B** shows the steps that were taken in the struggle against malaria.

Yellow fever, another infectious disease, was tracked down with as much courage and determination as was malaria. In 1900 many American soldiers in Cuba died of the disease. Walter Reed headed an army commission to find out about it. Two doctors allowed themselves to be bitten by mosquitoes to see if they carried yellow fever. One of the doctors died of the disease. Three volunteers then slept in sheets taken from the beds where people had died of yellow fever. They did not catch the disease. This proved that mosquitoes carried the disease. Again, as with malaria, measures could now be taken to prevent it.

Diseases like malaria and yellow fever have now been almost completely wiped out. This could not have happened without international cooperation (**D**).

B The fight against malaria

1870s Patrick Manson (1844-1922) was investigating elephantiasis in China and discovered that it was caused by worms blocking channels in the body. The worms in the blood were only active at night. Manson persuaded a Chinese volunteer to be bitten by a mosquito. The mosquito was cut open immediately afterwards and Manson found tiny parasites inside its stomach.

1880 Charles Leveran was an army commander. His men were dying of malaria and he managed to discover the parasite in their blood stream which was causing it.

1894/5 Manson met Ross (a London doctor) and suggested that Ross study mosquitoes in India to see if he could discover which ones or which species cause malaria.

1897 Ross discovered the species of mosquito which carry the malaria parasites.

1898 Sambon and Low (two of Manson's assistants) spent two months in the malaria-infested swamps near Rome, always returning at night to a mosquito-proof hut. They did not catch the disease.

1900 Manson allowed his own son to be bitten by a malaria-carrying mosquito and his son caught the disease. This proved finally that the disease is carried by the mosquito and passed on when the mosquito bites someone.

1950s Preventive methods were how used. Mosquito nets, creams and special clothes were invented. Insecticides like DDT were sprayed on the mosquito breeding grounds. This was largely the work of the World Health Organization.

After the Second World War in 1945, the United Nations Organization was set up. Its main aim was to prevent war happening again. One of the organizations that the UNO set up in 1948 was the World Health Organization (WHO).

With jet travel, diseases that might have taken years to cross the world during the nineteenth century can now cover the same distance in a matter of hours. WHO has managed to get international agreement to set up quarantine regulations to stop this. It has set up a centre

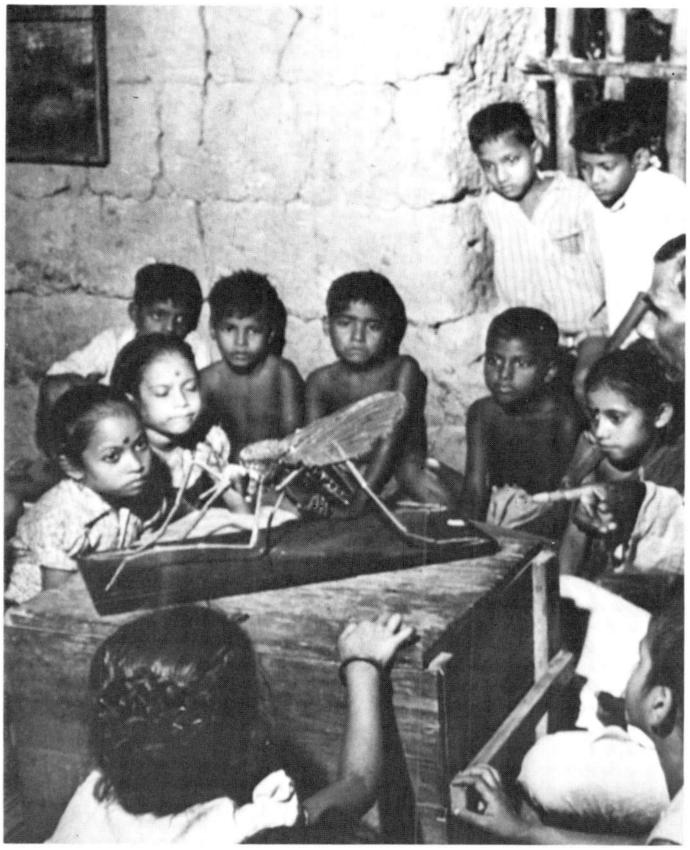

C A group of Indian children study a model of a malaria-carrying mosquito.

to gather statistics about world health, it sends teachers to under-developed countries, advises countries how to set up public health facilities and helps fight infectious diseases (see **C** and **E**).

D International health and humanitarian treaties and organizations
1851 *Congress of Paris* 12 European nations met to discuss methods of disease control. Nothing was settled but at least a start had been made. **1862** *A Memory of Solferino* by Jean Henri Dunant was published, describing the suffering from injury and disease of French soldiers in the war between France and Austria. It brought about; **1864** *The Geneva Convention* 16 European countries agreed to give protection to all injured soldiers on the battlefield. The Red Cross was the sign that was used to show where the injured were, so that the sides fighting each other would avoid that spot. **1902** *Pan American Sanitary Bureau* set up in Washington. **1948** *World Health Organization* set up as part of the United Nations.

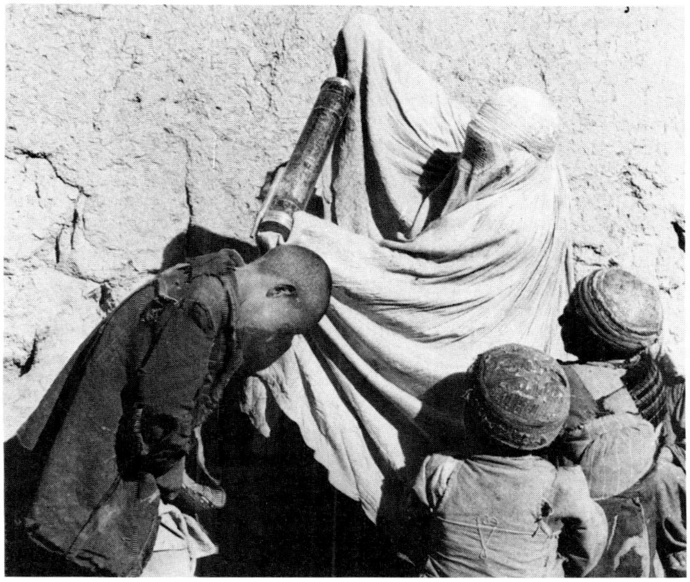

E A boy is doused with insecticide to get rid of external parasites in Afghanistan. This was part of a delousing campaign first organized by WHO.

??????????????????

1 Look at **A.** What were the three main causes of death in Britain between 1956 and 1966? Explain why they are different from those in the nineteenth century (see chapters 19, 25, 26).

2 Show in a chart like the one below how each of the following contributed to the eradication of infectious disease: Edward Jenner, Louis Pasteur, Joseph Lister, Edwin Chadwick, Patrick Manson, Charles Leveran, Ross, Sambon and Low, Manson's son, Walter Reed, WHO. Refer back to chapters 16, 17, 18, 19, 26 and 31.

Edward Jenner	Discovered vaccination could prevent smallpox
Louis Pasteur	
etc	

3 Look at **B.** Imagine it is 1900 and you are Patrick Manson's son. Write a report describing the experiment your father has just carried out and what you think it proves. You will have to mention the other experiments that have gone on before. You should mention: experiments on elephantiasis, identifying the malaria parasite; experiment to prove that mosquitoes carry malaria.

4 Imagine you are using the model shown in **C** to teach the children how to avoid catching malaria. Write down what you would say to them.

32 Penicillin and Other Drugs

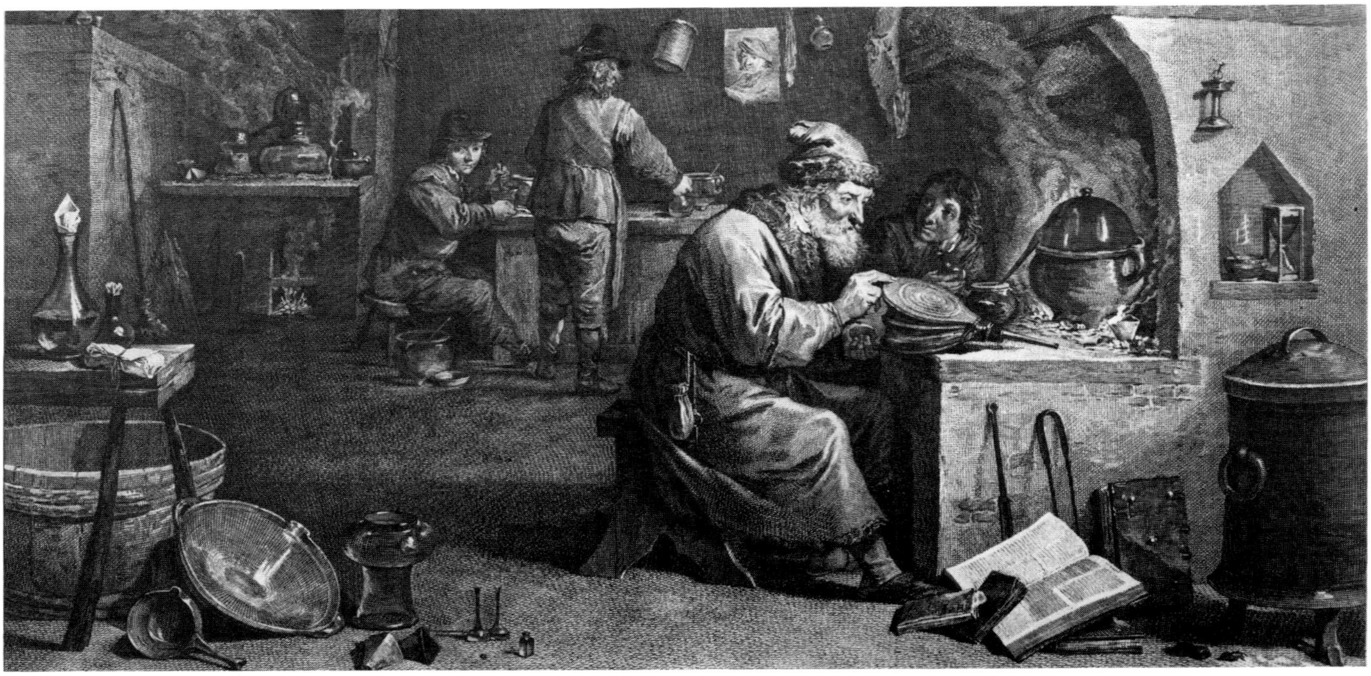

A An alchemist's laboratory in 1650. For thousands of years people had worked in rooms like these, trying to produce drugs and potions that might ease pain and cure diseases.

B Alexander Fleming in his laboratory in 1928

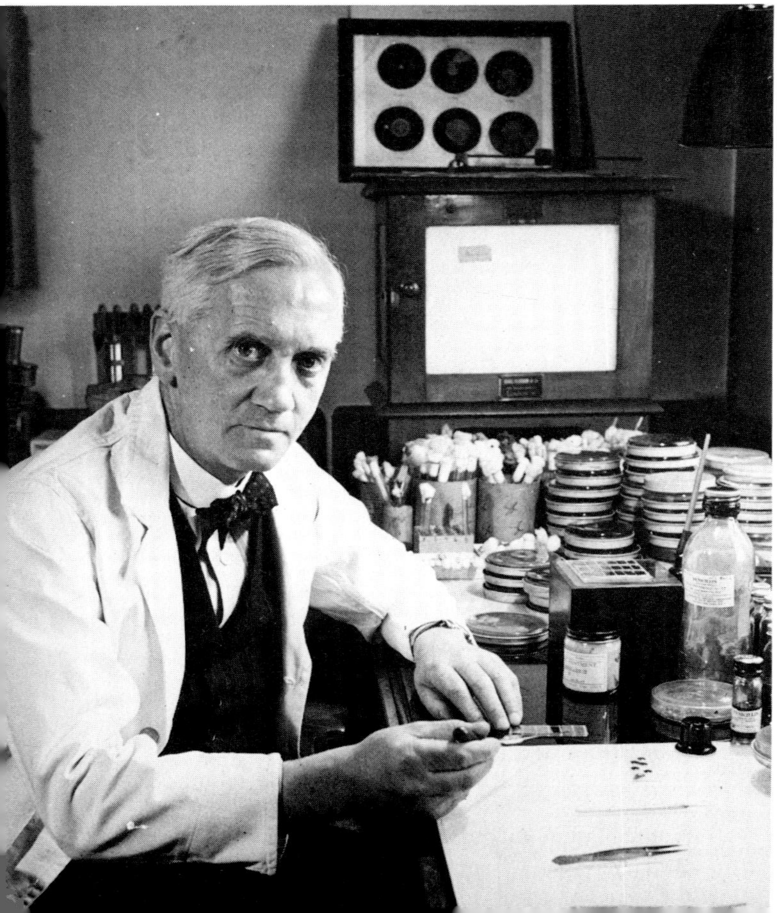

How many different drugs or medicines do you think you have taken since you were born? It is impossible for you to know. You will probably have taken aspirin for a headache. Ask your parents what sort of things you were given as a baby. There have been people, like those shown in **A**, making drugs for thousands of years, but it was not until giant chemical industries started to manufacture drugs on a large scale that many were on sale for all to buy in chemist's shops. This was not until the twentieth century.

Penicillin was the first of the so-called 'wonder drugs' because it killed off many different kinds of bacteria that caused disease. Alexander Fleming (**B**) discovered the drug by accident. He had seen how soldiers during the First World War (1914-18) died because of infection. In 1928 Fleming was growing a colony of bacteria when he noticed that some mould had grown on it. He also saw that all round the mould the bacteria he had been growing was dying off. He grew some more of this mould (known as penicillium notatum) and found that it killed many different bacteria. **C** is taken from Fleming's own account of the discovery:

❛ *The very first stage in the discovery of penicillin was due to a stroke of good fortune . . . There are thousands of different moulds and there are thousands of different bacteria . . . To begin with, all the manufacture was done in bottles . . . until a means of growing the mould in tanks was devised, but you cannot simply put it into a tank and expect good moulds. It grows on the top and you get a poor yield. It likes plenty of air so you have to blow in air and keep the fluid moving, and you have to blow in air without microbes – that is not easy. It was difficult chemical engineering but eventually they overcame the difficulties. This was one of the great advances made by Americans towards large-scale production and penicillin was soon being made in thousand gallon tanks, which not only saved labour but brought down the cost of production.* ❞ (**C**)

It was not until 1942 that penicillin was mass produced. The outbreak of the Second World War in 1939 meant that there was a need for the drug in large quantities. In 1941, the USA entered the war and their government gave large sums of money to American firms to produce penicillin because it could be used to stop infection spreading from wounds caused in battle. By the end of the war, penicillin had saved countless lives.

Chemotherapy is the treatment of disease by chemical substances. This technique had really got off the ground when Paul Ehrlich's team discovered Salvarsan 606 in 1910 (see chapter 30). Penicillin is just one example of how chemistry has helped medical progress. There are many others (**E**).

E	**New drugs and pills**
1803-19	Chemists begin to isolate chemicals from plants which can be used against disease
1819	Iodine first used
1820	Quinine used against malaria
1885	Amyl nitrate used for treatment of heart disease – angina
1898	Barbitone used as a sedative – the first barbiturate
1899	Aspirin sold in shops
1910	Ehrlich discovers salvarsan – the first 'magic bullet'
1911-12	Vitamins proved to be in food, and their importance understood
1921	Banting and Best discovered insulin. It helps cure diabetes (too much sugar in the blood system)
1928	Alexander Fleming discovers penicillin
1932	Prontosil in use, an effective drug against bacteria
1938	M & B 69s (named after May and Baker, the British firm which produced it) available. It helps to combat pneumonia, boils and wound infections. It was a sulphonamide drug prepared from a chemical dye. By 1942, 3,000 such drugs were helping to cure diseases such as meningitis, tonsilitis, scarlet fever and leprosy. Vitamins now given in pill form
1942	Penicillin mass-produced in the United States

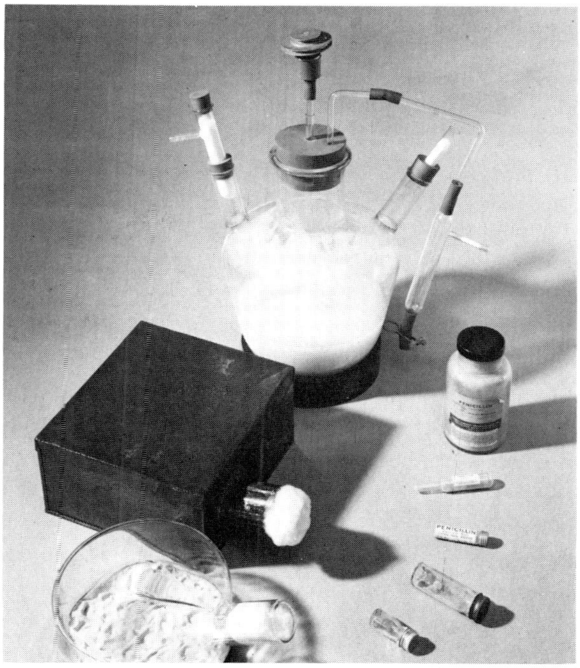

D Specimens of early penicillin preparation

??????????????????

1 Look at **A** and **B** and complete the following chart:

	Alexandria 1650	**Fleming's Lab** 1928
Number of people in laboratory		
Apparatus		
Cleanliness		

2 Imagine that you were with Fleming at the moment he discovered penicillin. Describe what happened. What did Fleming do? What did Fleming notice? What did he think the mould might be able to do?

3 Look at **C** and the text of the chapter:
- **a** In what way was the discovery of penicillin an accident?
- **b** List two of the problems faced when trying to produce penicillin.
- **c** Who eventually solved the problems and why?

4 Find out the symptoms of the following diseases mentioned in the text and say how chemotherapy has helped to cure them: pneumonia, meningitis, tonsilitis, scarlet-fever, leprosy, scurvy, diabetes and rickets.

5 How has each of the following helped in the discovery and production of drugs?
- **a** Warfare
- **b** Government help
- **c** Large industrial companies

33 Doctors' Aids

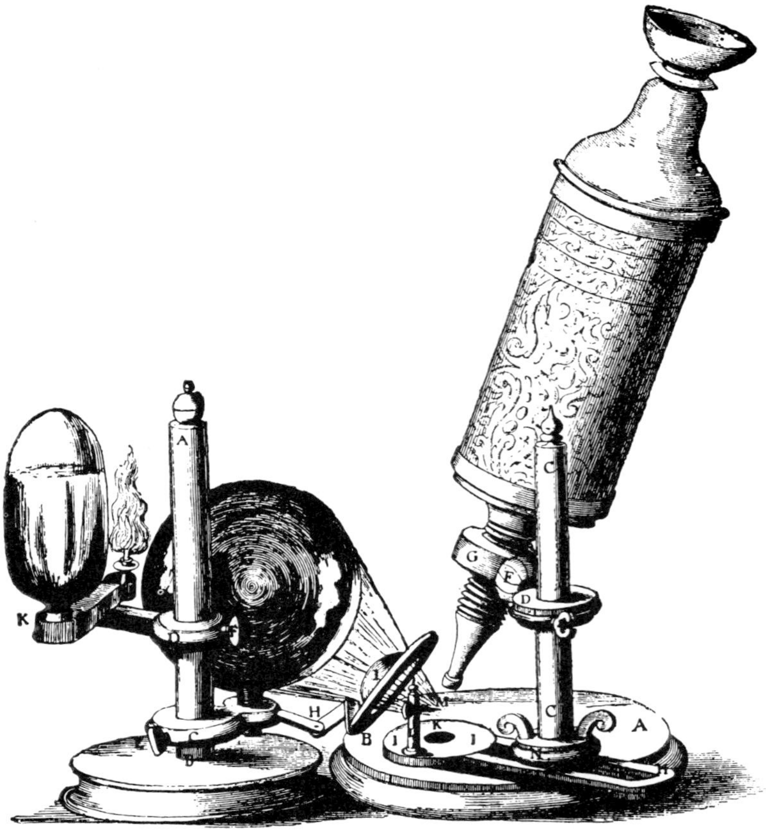

A Microscope made by the Englishman Robert Hooke in 1665

In 1661 King Charles II founded the Royal Society. Its aim was to use experiments to advance knowledge. The Royal Society tried to encourage scientific ways of looking at things. This way of thinking helped the progress of medicine.

Sanctorius (an Italian) had developed a thermometer by 1630. The microscope was developed by several people, including Malpighi (1628-94), Leeuwenhoeck (1632-1723) and Robert Hooke, an Englishman and member of the Royal Society, who invented the microscope shown in **A.**

René Laennec invented the first stethoscope in 1816 after realizing that he could hear a patient's heartbeat through a rolled-up piece of cardboard. Over the years the stethoscope developed into the modern version with two ear tubes.

The Industrial Revolution (see chapter 19) caused a growth in technology and this was the source of many new aids for doctors. Karl Ludwig (1816-95) invented a kymograph, which was a machine that used a pen to trace breathing and blood pressure. Poiseuille invented an instrument for measuring blood pressure.

The discovery of X-rays by Wilhelm Roentgen in 1895 has been one of the most important aids for doctors in the twentieth century (see **B**).

X-rays pass through the skin but not the bone and so X-ray photographs can show where a bone is fractured. They can also be used to cure warts and blemishes on the skin and recent research shows that they can help to cure cancer. The artifical kidney machine (**C**) and iron lung machine are two more recent inventions. Surgeons can also replace hearts, kidneys and corneas of eyes. They can fit artificial limbs.

B This is a photograph of a computerized tomographic scanner. The machine uses X-rays to photograph slices through any part of the human body.

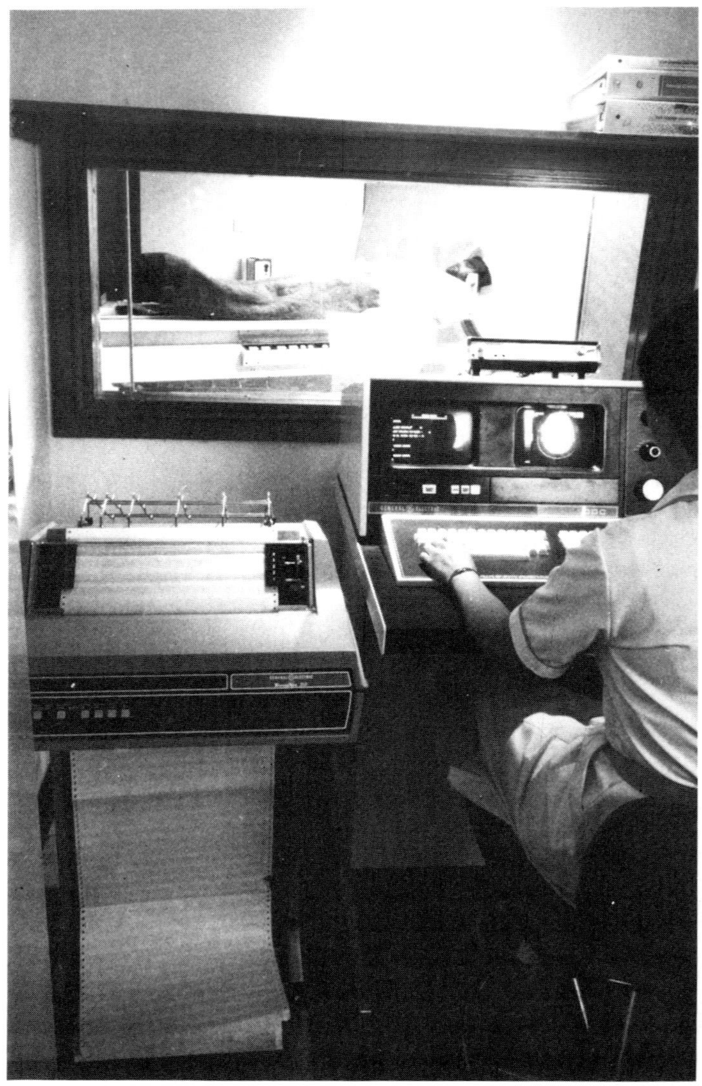

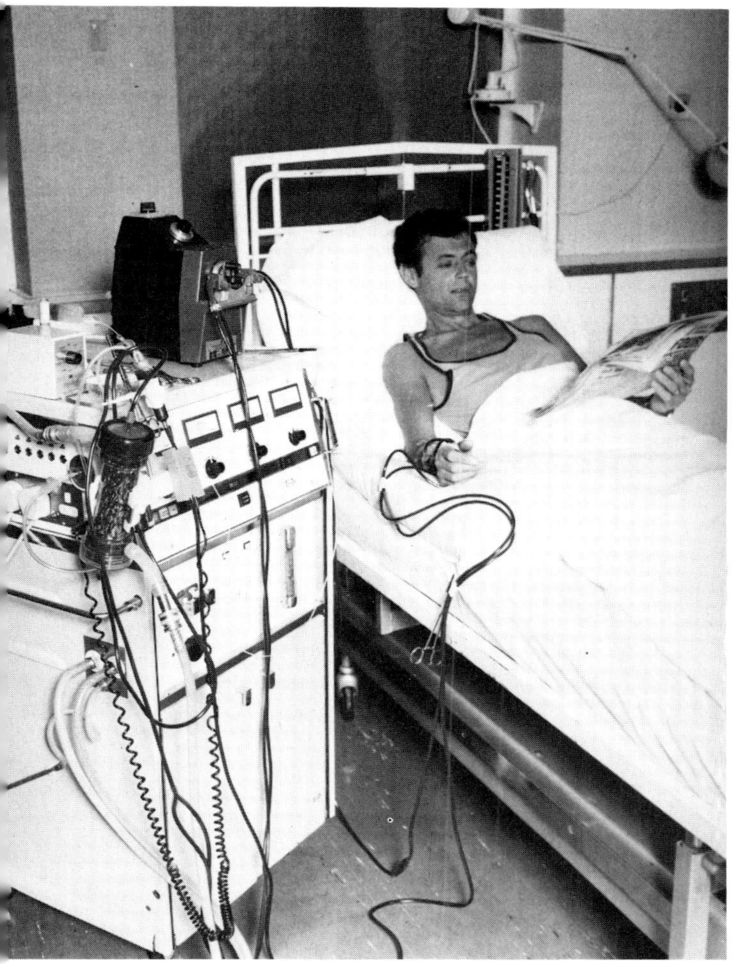

C A kidney machine

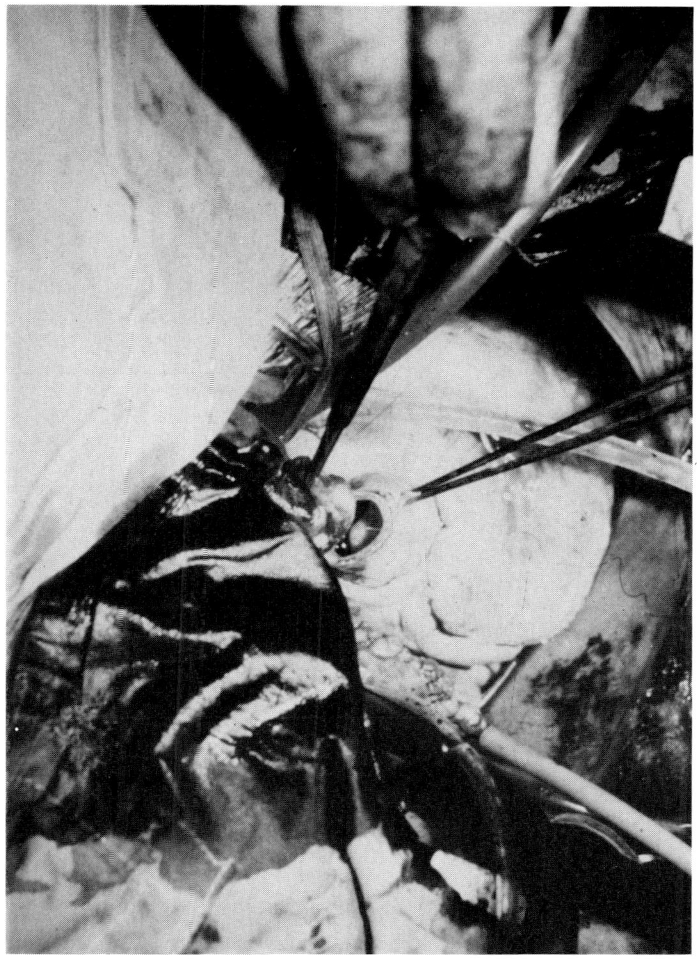

E A heart transplant operation.

Dr Christian Barnard here describes the first heart transplant operation carried out in 1967:

❛ *To achieve this we used all the techniques of modern medicine to spy on the hidden interior of the human body. Kidney function was checked by measuring its urine output . . . the heart pattern was plotted by an electrocardiagram. The lungs were X-rayed . . . blood chemistry was checked in the laboratory . . . We took swabs from the skin, nose, throat, mouth and rectum. We also washed* (the patient) *continually with an antiseptic solution and an antibiotic ointment was put up his nose. Room 207, where he was to be nursed after the operation, was fumigated; its walls and floor plus all cracks and corners were washed with disinfectant. Every utensil in the room was boiled. All members of staff who were to look after the patient had their noses, throats and rectums also studied.*

We needed two teams of men and women. One would hold in life some vital organs of the donor, while the other prepared Louis Washinsky (the patient who was to receive the heart). *A single error on either side would collapse the whole operation.* ❜ **(D)**

?????????????????

1 a What is the importance of X-rays? Who discovered them?

b This instrument enabled doctors to see bacteria for the first time and to examine minute parts of the body such as the capillaries. It was developed by Malpighi and Leeuwenhoeck. What is it?

c This aid for doctors was invented by René Laennec and enables doctors to listen clearly to the heart beat. Draw a picture of it as it looks today.

2 Name some other aids for doctors not mentioned in question **1** above and say how they helped doctors and surgeons.

3 Look at **D**. Give four ways in which it shows an attempt to achieve aseptic surgery.

4 How has surgery improved in the past 200 years? Tell its story as if you were talking to medical students.

34 The Welfare State

In a *Welfare State* the government looks after the welfare of the people instead of expecting them to do so themselves. The Romans had partly done this when they set up a public health system for all citizens (see chapter 7). But in Britain, even as late as the nineteenth century, governments followed a policy known as 'laissez-faire'. This is a French phrase meaning 'to leave alone'. These governments thought that it was not their job to interfere with people's lives unless they really had to. This is one reason why it took so long for measures like the Public Health Act of 1875 (see chapter 26) to come into force. **A** shows some of the landmarks in the growth of the Welfare State in Britain:

A	**Landmarks in the growth of the Welfare State**
1902	Midwives Act. Midwives had to be properly trained and registered.
1906	Free school meals introduced for poor children.
1907	School medical inspections began.
1908	Old Age Pensions Act. Free old age pensions.
1909	Town Planning Act. Back-to-back houses forbidden.
1911	National Health Insurance Act. Unemployed men could draw money if they were out of work through sickness.
1919 **1923** **1924**	Subsidized Housing Acts. Local Authorities built council houses.
1942	Beveridge Report recommended National Insurance Scheme where unemployed could draw money for an indefinite period of time.
1945	Family Allowance Act gave money to families for each child.
1948	National Health Service set up.

B shows how some poor people survived in Britain in the early 1900s:

❛ *When I was a child, there was no National Health Service. People paid into sick clubs. Miners had 2d a week stopped from their wages to pay for doctors if they were ill. Surgeries were held in someone's sitting room if the doctors had no spare room. They had just a few bottles to make up medicine. This had to cost no more than 2d.*

Even so, most people could not afford the doctors' fees and so they treated themselves. For sprains and bruises we fomented wild plants like comfrey and dog standard. For confinements we had to pay the doctor £1.1s or a neighbour could help out. That was all right if there were no complications. My husband's father used to burn camphor on a hot shovel and blow it about the room when my husband and his four sisters and three brothers were coughing.

I fell off a wall and hurt my right knee . . . (the pain) *later settled in my hip. The doctor said I had hip-joint disease and wanted to send me to hospital. My mother did not want me to go so the doctor said he would treat me at home but we must pay 3s 6d each time he came. He would paint my hip with iodine one week and the next he would put a plaster on it. This made a big blister come up which he then pricked to let the fluid out. I did not walk for almost a year. I have often thought what a sacrifice my parents must have made to pay for the doctor when my father's wage was only one sovereign and a shilling a week.* ❜ **(B)**

From Schools Council History, Medicine Through Time, Book III

Slowly British governments came to accept that a better method of looking after the poor was needed. One of the first government ministers to provide one was David Lloyd George. He introduced the National Insurance Act in 1911 (see **C**). Many people were against the act. Doctors did not like it because they thought they would be too rushed to do the job properly, if they had too many poor people to deal with. Lloyd George got over this opposition by paying each doctor more money for each patient he saw.

After the First World War in 1918, thousands of houses were needed to provide homes for the soldiers who

C Government leaflet issued in 1911 explains how the new National Insurance scheme will work.

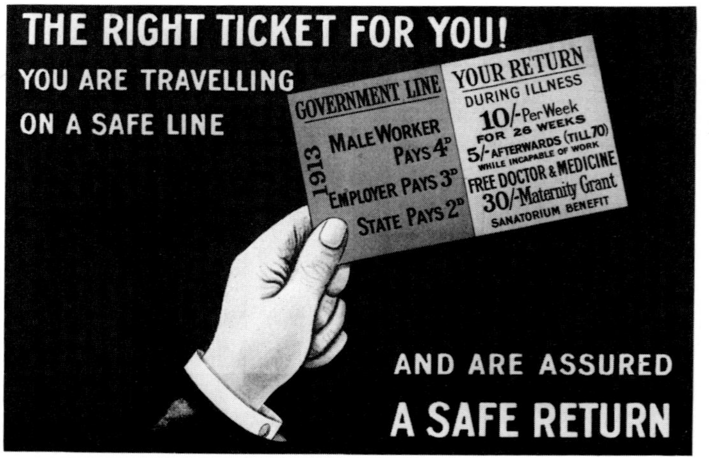

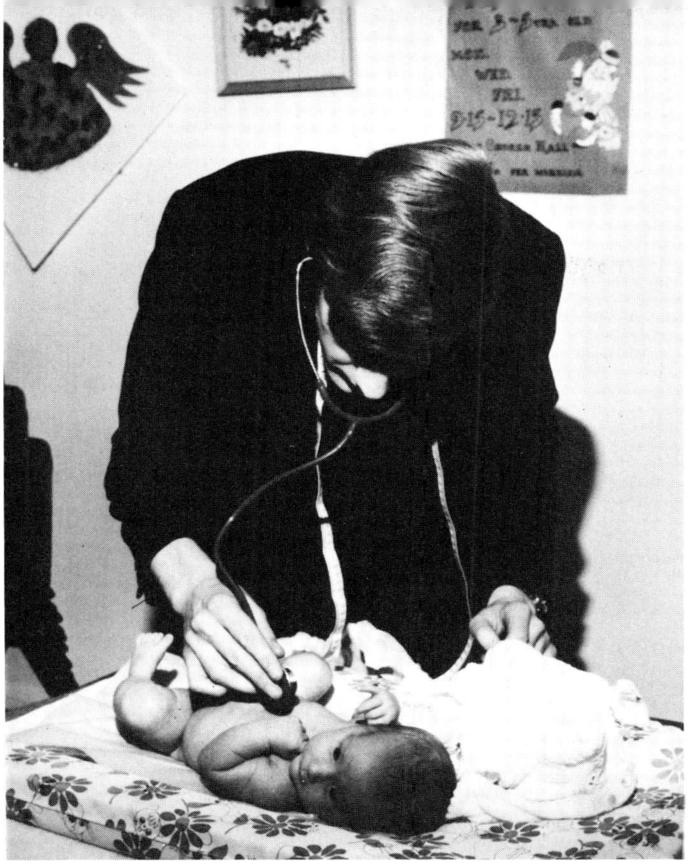

D A post-natal clinic set up by the National Health Service

returned. During the 1920s many council houses were built and this was one very important aspect of the Welfare State. It meant that the government realized it was its job to see that people had decent houses. The real breakthrough in terms of medical care, though, came as a result of the Second World War of 1939-45.

In 1939 the Health Service was still based on Lloyd George's act of 1911. Wives and children of insured workers could still not get free medical treatment. The war forced the government to make changes. A survey in 1938 showed that there was a shortage of hospital beds. This would mean that there would not be enough beds for people hurt in bombing raids. The government provided the money that was needed to improve the hospital facilities. Doctors and surgeons were obliged to leave the rich areas of the south and work in the poorer industrial areas farther north.

In 1945 the National Health Service Act was passed. A whole range of medical services was provided free of charge. A national system of General Practitioners (GPs) was set up. Everyone could consult a doctor anywhere quickly without having to pay. Health centres (see **D**) were set up. These were places where groups of doctors gathered together to offer a full range of medical services in one building. Yet in 1946 two out of every three doctors were against the setting up of the Health Service because they said it meant they were not free to work for themselves any more. On 5 July 1948, the day the Health Service officially came into being, *The Daily Mirror* reported:

❛ *THE DAY IS HERE For years the reformers of all parties have tried to safeguard the aged, the poor and the sick. Much has been done – much more than in any other country. But always you wanted greater protection against misfortune. You wanted the state to accept larger responsibility for the individual citizen who served it faithfully. You wanted Social Security, from this day hence, you have it.* ❜ **(E)**

Nearly one twentieth of a total salary goes to the government to pay for National Insurance. This money would help to provide sick pay if you fell ill and could not work. Some of the tax would go towards helping to pay for the National Health Service.

??????????????????

1 Look at **A** and **B,** and then compare how you might be looked after today with how a schoolboy or girl in 1900 was looked after. Mention under headings *Then* and *Now*: medical care and inspections at school, visits to the doctors, medicines, payment for treatment, the Health Service.

2 Which three acts listed in **A** do you think would have had most effect on the British people? Explain your answer.

3 Why did doctors oppose:
- **a** The National Health Insurance Act 1911 and
- **b** The National Health Service 1948?

4 Describe how each of the following has helped to bring about a welfare state in Britain:
- **a** *Two world wars:* Mention the homeless after World War One and how World War Two showed that the government had to do something.
- **b** *Government action:* Mention the Public Health Act 1875 (see chapter 26), other government acts before World War Two (see **A**) and the setting up of the National Health Service.

5
- **a** Look at **B** and then list all the things people did in the early 1900s to look after themselves that people would probably not have to do today.
- **b** Name any three benefits that the National Health Service has brought about.
- **c** Are there any ways in which you think the National Health Service could be improved?
- **d** What do you think of the idea that private paying patients should be allowed to have beds in a National Health hospital?

35 Medicine and the Third World

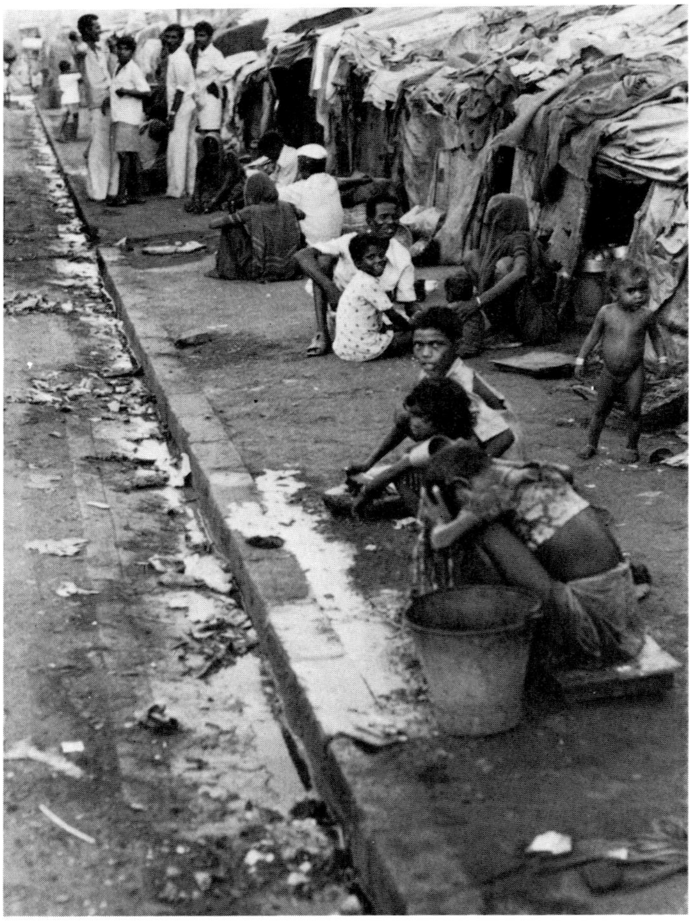

A Street dwellers in Bombay, India

Look at **A** and **B**. These sources show some of the reasons why people in developing countries in the Third World contract more diseases than people in Britain. They are not as well fed and they cannot live in good houses or near clean water. We tend to take clean water for granted in Britain and most of us don't really realise what would happen to us if we couldn't get clean water easily.

C is written by a scientist who specialises in water-borne diseases. She describes how difficult it is to prevent children in Ghana catching diseases from dirty water:

‘*Children living in areas with inadequate water supplies and sanitation are liable to infection with many of the water borne diseases. If they live in a tsetse* (disease carrying insect) *belt they are liable to catch sleeping sickness. If they farm in a valley or fish in a river infected with similium damnosum* (a bacteria present in infected water) *they are liable to become infected and perhaps become blind ... There is no doubt at all that bad sanitation contributes immensely to the dangers to which children are exposed. Water will always have a special fascination for children. Sneaking down to the river to bathe, swim and generally splash about is perhaps the brightest activity in the otherwise dreary life of many rural children. But the threat of disease will continue until women, children and entire communities come to understand the importance of safe water and good sanitation.*’ (**C**)

B Some statistics comparing Third World and Developed countries

Country	Life expectancy	Deaths per 1000 in first year after birth	Population per doctor	% of Population with safe water supply	Daily food intake in calories
Upper Volta	43	263	49810	25	1875
India	52	125	3620	33	2021
Indonesia	53	120	13640	12	2272
Britain	73	14	750	100	3336

Figures from World Bank World Development Report, 1981.

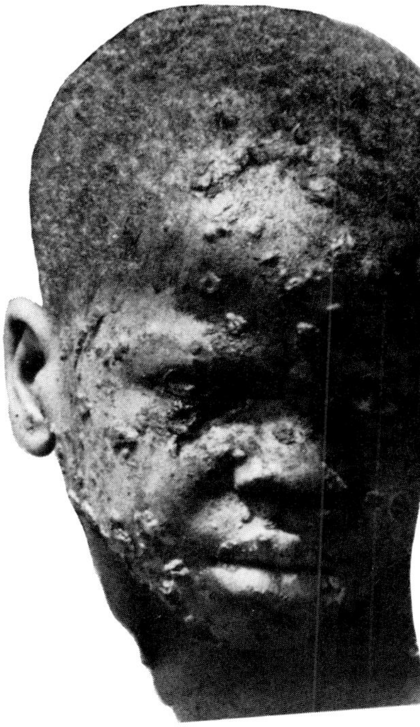

C Child suffering from *Yaws*.

You might be tempted, cruelly, to say 'Well, it's their own faults then, they ought to know better and not use the water'. But a closer look at **B** will show you that many children do not have access to clean water, so they have no choice. And if you can't believe that children would willingly play in infected water, just think how many times recently you or your friends have bathed in the sea off the coast of Britain – these very waters have recently been declared by the EEC to be among the dirtiest in the world.

Besides a lack of clean drinking water, there are four other major reasons why there are so many medical problems in the Third World.

The ignorance factor has already been hinted at in **C**. By ignorance we don't mean that the people themselves are stupid or less intelligent than others, we mean that they simply have not yet discovered what actually causes disease. Organisations like the *United Nations* and the *World Health Organisation* are trying to educate Third World people in the techniques of disease prevention, but it takes a long time and it costs a lot of money.

Poor sanitation is another major cause of disease in these countries. **A** shows an example of this, where dirty water is situated near to drinking water. Again, it is not stupidity that causes this situation; the people just don't have money to spend on the technology needed to improve drainage and sewage disposal, things we take for granted in Britain.

Bad living conditions cause disease and poor health for the same reasons mentioned above.

Poor food means that people are not strong or healthy enough to fight off many of the diseases they encounter.

'We do a lot to help these countries, isn't it about time they did something to help themselves?' This is a question you will often hear people ask. It is really just an excuse to try and cover up the fact that we in the Developed World really don't do enough to help struggling countries. There are many examples of the ways developing countries have used scarce resources to encourage better health care themselves. Look at extract **D** taken from GEO Magazine, 1985.

❛In Tami Nadu in India, they began by setting up hospitals to cure sick people. Then they set up teams of qualified doctors and midwives to tour the villages but soon discovered that these hospital trained staff were not on the same wavelength as the village people. Much of what they taught was too expensive or too impractical. So they started recruiting village girls and training them as health workers Within two years they had twenty-two mobile teams visiting every village in the region every two weeks. Eventually they moved towards having permanent health workers in every village. After a few months training, these village doctors can recognise most of the more common diseases and help people to prevent them from spreading. The very best workers become community organisers and help the villagers to build their own clinics and to train more people to work in them . . . This programme is typical of those used by poor communities all over the world.❜ (**D**)

??????????????????

1 **a** Using sources **A–D**, make a list of all the causes of poor health in the Third World.
b Pick one of the causes you have listed in **a**. Discuss and write down all the things that could be done to remove this cause of disease.
c What are the major problems that have to be overcome before you could put into practice the ideas you have just written down in **b**?

2 How would you persuade the mother of one of the children described in **C** that she should not allow her child to play in the river? Write down a possible conversation between the mother and you. You could do this with a friend, each of you taking one of the characters.

3 Which of the pieces of evidence in this chapter tells you most about medicine in the Third World and what does it tell you?

36 Women in Medicine

A father is driving his son to school when they are involved in a serious accident and taken by ambulance to the local hospital. As the boy is about to be operated upon, the surgeon suddenly cries out, 'Oh no! That's my son.'

How can this be? There is a good chance that if you had tried to work out the answer to this question before reading the rest of this chapter, it would have taken you a long time to come to the conclusion that the surgeon was the boy's mother. We don't immediately think of women as being surgeons; we regard it as a man's job. Similarly, we generally think of nurses as being women when in fact 5% of nurses are men. There is no reason why women should not be surgeons, nor why men should not be nurses.

Stereotyping is the word we use for deciding beforehand what we expect certain people to be like. In the history of medicine, women have often been stereotyped as the gentler, more caring sex and encouraged to perform certain jobs or roles, usually the supportive roles rather than the creative ones. Many of you might argue that the title of chapter one of this book does just that: who is to say that women were any less important than men in the development of medicine in prehistoric times? What might have been a fairer title for chapter one?

Apart from Florence Nightingale (chapter 24), women have rarely been specifically mentioned in this book. This is not because women did not play a significant part in the development of medicine. Over the centuries, restrictive attitudes towards women taking up medicine as a career meant that few women were able to do so, except as nurses, and even fewer were mentioned by historians. It is very difficult to assess the part women actually did play, and even more difficult to say the part they *might* have played if only they had been given more encouragement.

B 1897. Male students at the university of Cambridge protest against the admission of women onto degree courses. They were successful and degrees were not given to women at Cambridge until 1922.

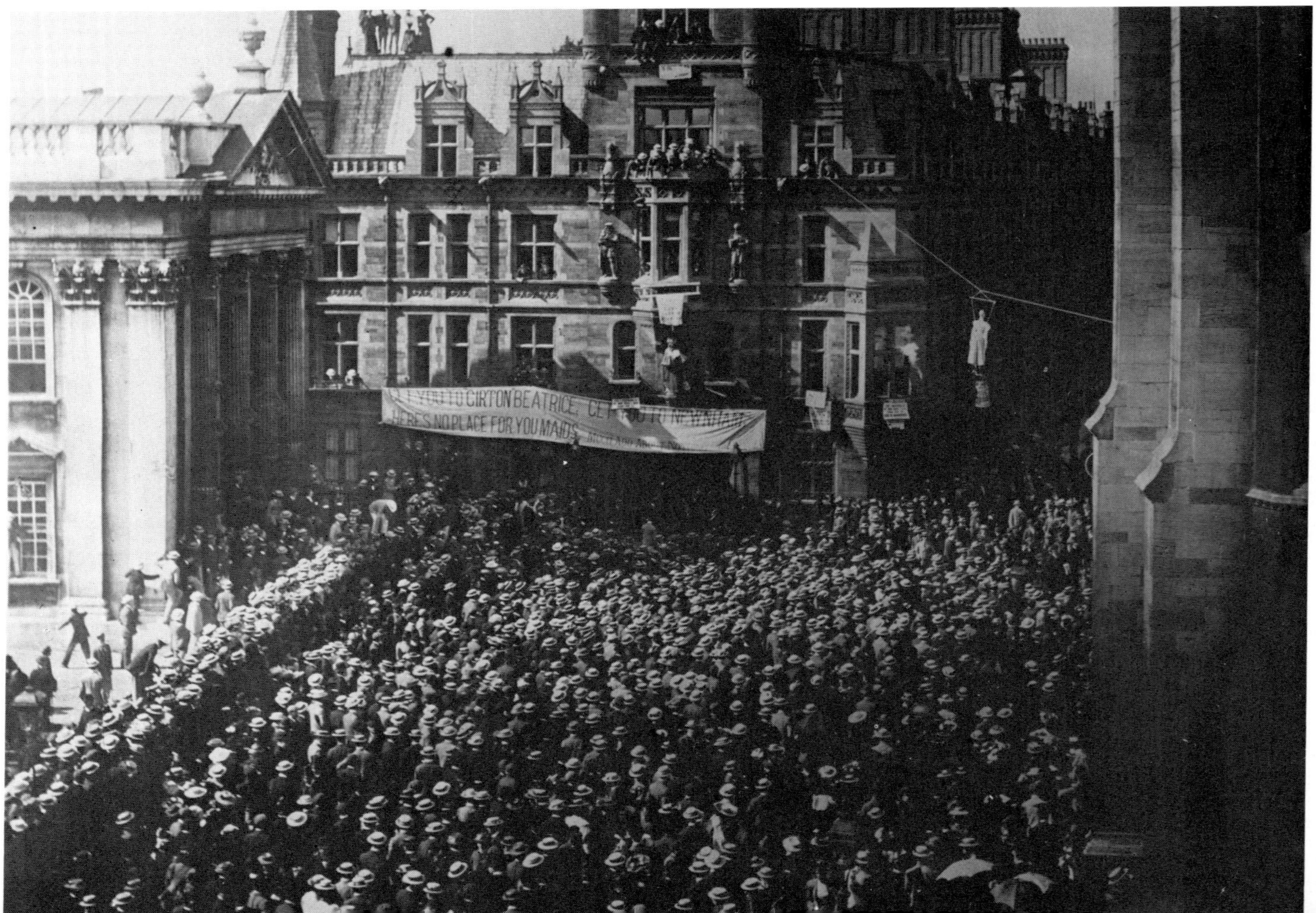

If it is difficult today for women to be accepted in the top jobs in medicine, just imagine how much more difficult it was for women in the past. **A** is taken from a report written in 1857 and is representative of the views about training for nurses held by many surgeons in the 19th century:

❛*Nurses are in much the same position as housemaids and require little teaching beyond that of poultice-making which is easily acquired, the enforcement of cleanliness and attention to the patients' wants. This proposed hospital nurse training scheme has not met with the support of the medical profession.*❜ (**A**)

B shows how much opposition there was at the end of the 19th century to women becoming educated at universities. Even Florence Nightingale (see chapter 24) faced great opposition from her own father and from society (male society especially) when she tried to improve standards of nursing care.

However, courageous women like Florence Nightingale paved the way for other women to make their mark in the history of medicine. Elizabeth Garrett Anderson was another (**C**). She read the following poem in *Punch* magazine in 1849 and decided that she would try to become a doctor:

❛*Young ladies all, of every clime,*
Especially of Britain
Who wholly occupy your time
in novels or in knitting,
Whose highest skill is but to play,
Sing, dance or French to clack well,
Reflect on the example, pray,
Of excellent Miss Blackwell.❜ (**D**)

C Elizabeth Garrett Anderson

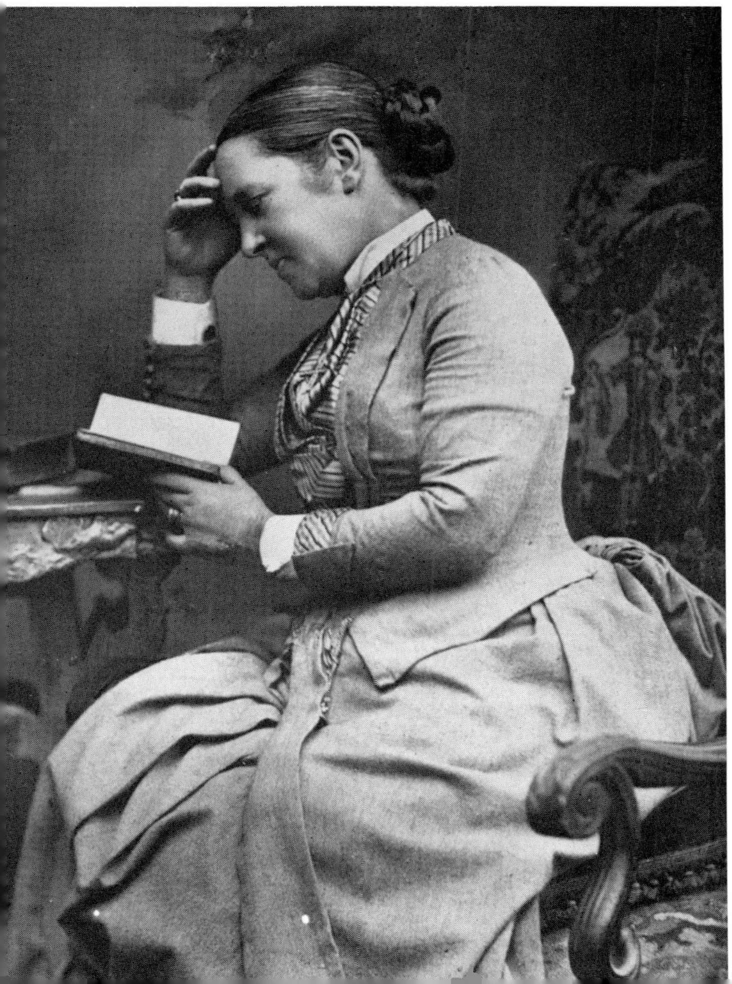

Miss Blackwell was American and the first woman in the world to become a doctor. Her father strongly opposed her at first, but eventually paid for her to have private lessons. First she trained as a nurse and listened in to lectures given to medical students. By 1858 she had passed all her exams but still could not become a doctor until the College of Physicians and the College of Surgeons allowed her to do so. They refused and, as we have seen, no British University would allow her to study medicine. So, she learnt French, studied in Paris, and, in 1870, became a Doctor of Medicine. Women have gained a great many more freedoms since that time, but these are too great to cover in a book about medicine. Florence Nightingale and Elizabeth Anderson are merely examples to show how courageous and determined women had to be to make any impact in the medical world. This is probably why there are so few famous women in medicine mentioned in the history books.

??????????????????

1 Why does the writer of **A** think it is unnecessary to train nurses? Does the writer of **D** hold the same opinion of women? Explain your answer.
2 Using all the information in this chapter, write a speech that the leader of the demonstration in **B** might have made explaining why women should not be admitted to Cambridge University.
3 Look back to chapter 21. Another famous woman made an important contribution to the development of medicine. Who was she and what contribution did she make?
4 Do a longer piece of writing explaining why women have found it so difficult to make significant contributions to the development of medicine until more recent years.

37 Technology and Medicine

Today, when you mention the word *technology* most of us think of computers or complicated electronic gadgets. But technology is really something much wider than this.

Technology is the way we use natural resources, materials and energy to control and change our lives. It doesn't matter whether these resources are complicated electronic gadgets like computers, simple things like a map to help us find our way, or a stretcher to carry us to an operating theatre.

Hard technology is the term which describes inventions or objects that help us in our lives (things like computers, calculators or washing machines).

Design technology (soft technology) is the use of other natural resources to solve problems, natural resources like common sense cures for illnesses or ways of organising groups of people so they work well together to solve problems. You might not immediately think of these things as *technology*, but they are, and both *hard* and *soft* technology have had an effect on the progress of medicine as the sources in this chapter show. Pictures **A**, **B** and **C** each show an example of a kind of technology that has had an effect on the progress of medicine. **D** is a description of a simple method used by Doctor Semmelweis in Hungary in the 1840s when he used existing technology to solve a problem in the maternity wards of the hospital where he worked. It was a practical method used to solve a practical problem, a technological way of working.

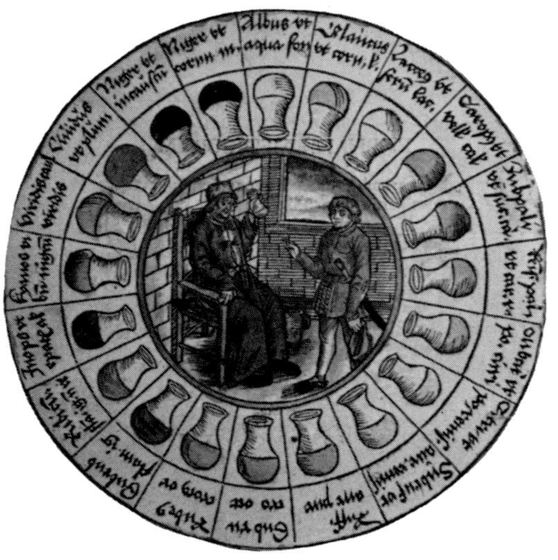

A Urine chart used by doctors in the Middle Ages. It helped doctors to classify the colour of a patient's urine and from this they hoped to be able to say what was wrong with the patient.

‘*In May 1847 he (Semmelweiss) asked his students to wash their hands in chlorinated lime water, and to scrub their fingernails with a handbrush before entering the ward. The death rate in this ward then stood at 12.4%. Within two months it fell to 1.27%.*’ (**D**)

From A Pictoral History of Medicine *by O Bettman*

Dr Christian Barnard (see chapter 33) described how all the modern technology available in 1967, when he carried out the first heart transplant operation, was needed to make the operation a success: (**E**)

B A printing press in the sixteenth century.

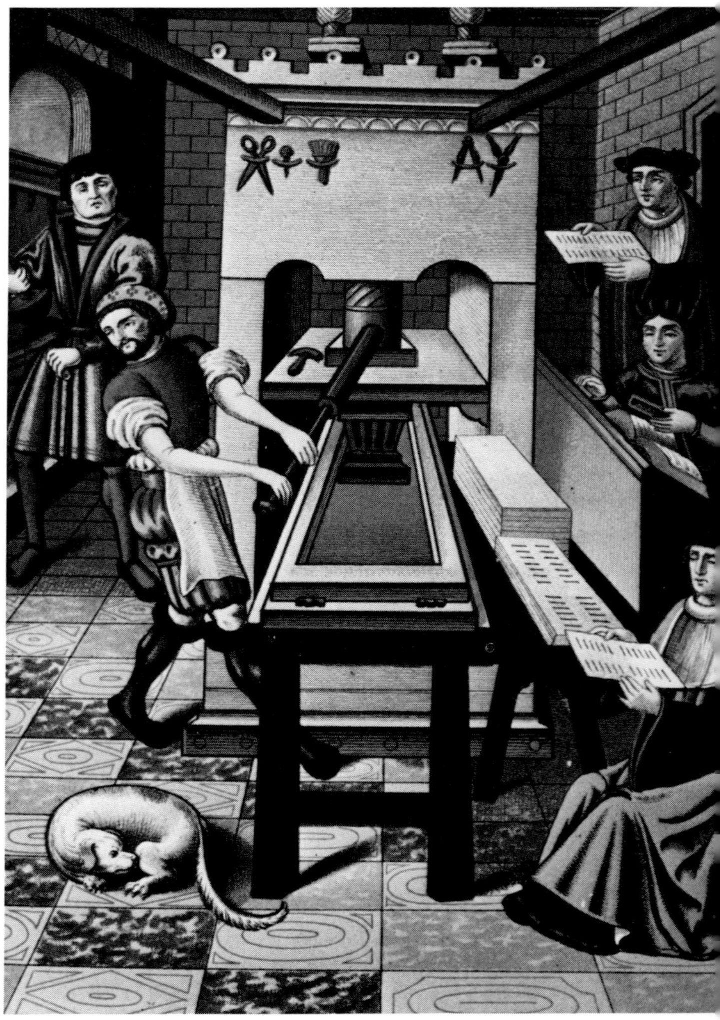

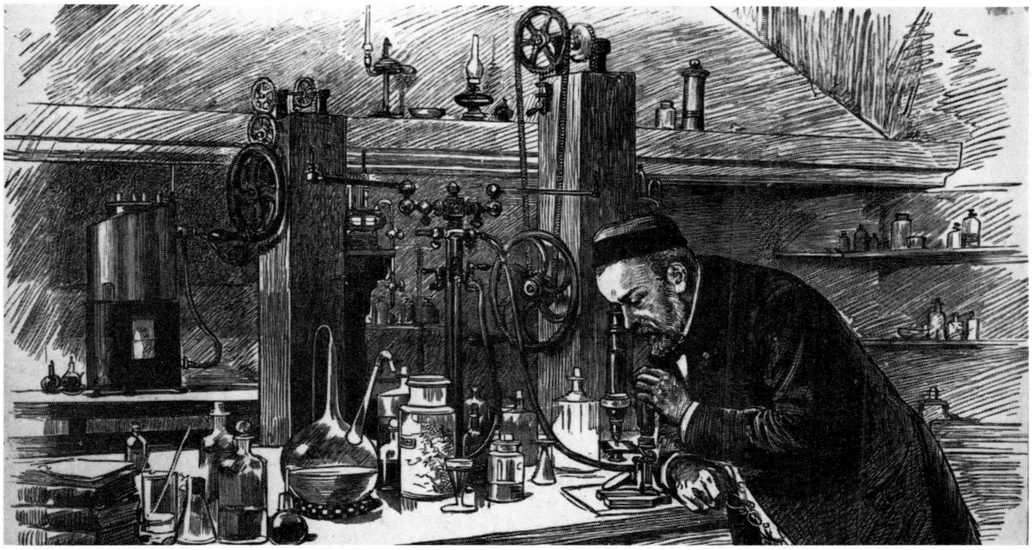

C An early microscope.

❛Kidney function was checked by measuring the urine output . . . The liver was studied through urine and blood analysis. The heart pattern was plotted by an electrocardiagram. The lungs were X-rayed . . . Blood chemistry was also checked in the laboratory . . . We also washed him continually with Phisohex, an antiseptic solution . . . and an antibiotic ointment was put up his nose to prevent organisms from accumulating there. Room 207 where he was to be nursed after the operation was fumigated, its walls and floor, plus all cracks and corners were washed with Phenolic disinfectant. Every utensil in the room was boiled. All members of staff who were to look after the patient had their noses, throats and rectums also studied.❜ **(E)**

But not all technological developments bring good or beneficial results. In 1988 the newspapers and television news broadcasts were full of reports like **F** about a drug that brought horrible deformity and death to thousands of arthritis sufferers.

PATIENT SUES OVER OPREN 'TESTS' A YEAR AFTER ALERT

A row flared yesterday over Opren 'tests' carried out in Britain more than a year after the drug's licence was taken away. Opren's licence was suspended in 1982 after side effects were reported in 3,563 arthritis patients, 83 of whom died. Eli Lilly, the manufacturers, has been widely criticised for offering 1,350 victims less than £1,600 each in compensation.

F From *The Daily Mail*, 25th April 1988.

??????????????????

1 Complete a chart like the one below, using all of the pieces of evidence in this chapter, to show which are examples of *hard technology* and *design technology*.

Evidence	Hard technology (brief explanation)	Design technology (brief explanation)
A	A urine chart; this is an invention used to solve a problem.	
B		

2 Which of the pieces of evidence about technology shown in this chapter do you think had the greatest effect on the progress of medicine? Explain your answer with examples.

3 Look at **E** and **F**. What criticisms could you make about the use of new technology in medicine using these sources only as examples? You might like to arrange your answer under the headings: Cost, Who loses out? Should people be used as guinea-pigs? Could the time and money be better spent trying to cure common illnesses?

4 Look back in this book and see how technology (in its widest sense) has effected the progress of medicine in each of the following periods: prehistoric times; the Roman period; the Renaissance; the 19th century.

38 War and its Effects on Medicine

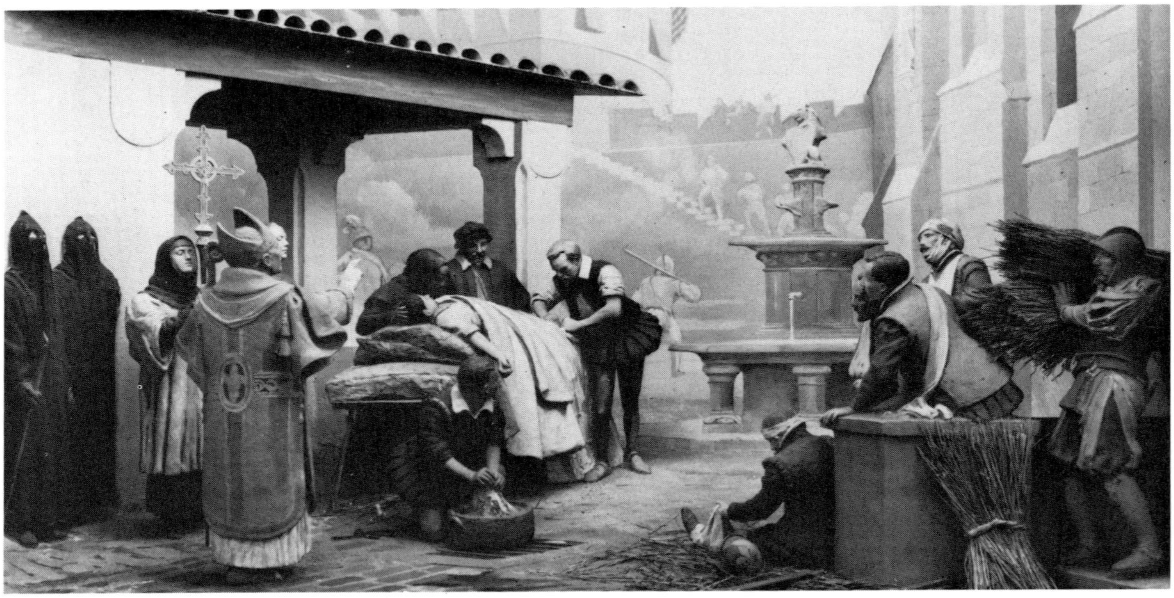

A Pare operating on a battlefield in the 16th Century

You are out on the school field. Without warning, an aeroplane drops a bomb, destroying the school and injuring your best friends. The person next to you has a wound that needs treating. Could you manage? You probably *would* think of something to do in these circumstances. Sometimes unforeseen events bring out the inventiveness in all of us. In many ways, war has speeded up progress in the medical world because people have been forced to find solutions to problems very quickly.

War is a terrible thing. People die, buildings are destroyed, and people suffer. Yet war has had some positive results. A glimpse at picture **A**, chapter 7 might help you to see how soldiers in Roman times had to learn how to deal with injuries quickly in order to get the troops fit enough to fight again on the battlefield.

Just as the Roman soldiers on page 14 had to try out new surgical techniques, so too did Ambroise Pare (see chapter 15) during the 16th century. Source **A** shows Pare operating on a soldier wounded in battle. You can see the hurried and makeshift conditions in which he had to work. Bad as these conditions were, they sometimes forced surgeons to develop important new methods as Pare himself explained in 1536:

❛*Wounds made of firearms (contain) poison because of the powder. For their cure (it is suggested that we need to) cauterise them with boiling oil or elder . . . Eventually my oil lacked* (thickened) *and I was constrained to apply in its place a digestive made of the yolks of eggs, oil of roses and turpentine.*❜ (**B**)

You may remember from chapter 15 that this treatment was a great success. But Pare had no way of knowing that it would be a success. The battle forced him to try out something new and he discovered a new technique for treating gunshot wounds by doing so.

Much of the work to improve standards of nursing done by Florence Nightingale might never have been done had she not been inspired to go to the Crimea and help out there (see chapter 24). The letter that prompted her to go was from Sidney Herbert (Secretary of State for War) and it shows clearly how the war prompted changes in nursing standards:

❛*Dear Miss Nightingale,*
You will have seen in the papers that there is a great shortage of nurses at Scutari, none but male nurses having ever been admitted to military hospitals. I receive numbers of offers from ladies to go out, but they have no idea of what a hospital is, nor of the nature of the duties.

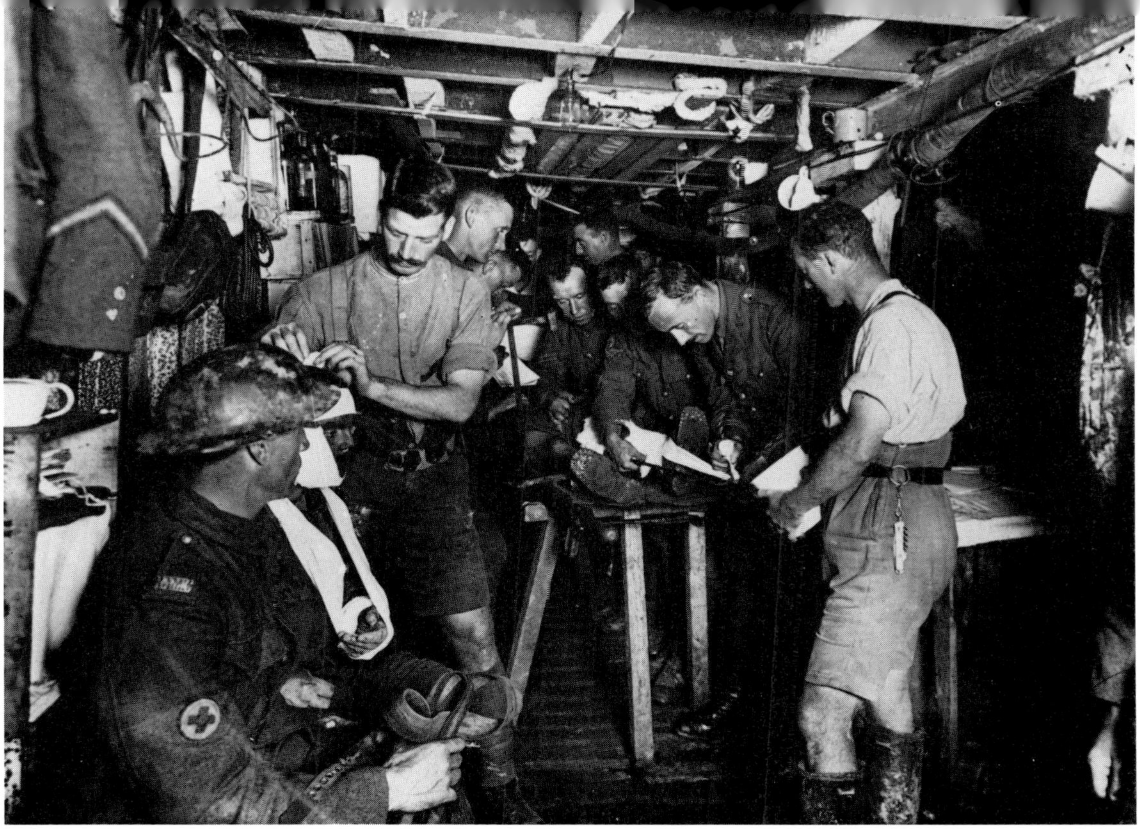

D A field hospital in World War One

Would you listen to the request to go and superintend the whole thing? I know you will come to a wise decision.❜ (**C**)

Later, in 1864, *The Geneva Convention* was signed by representatives of 16 European countries to protect all injured soldiers on the battlefield. A red cross was used to mark where the hospitals were, and all countries agreed not to fire on a station showing this sign.

You might think by looking at **D** that surgery during warfare had not improved very much since Roman times. But the two world wars this century have brought about a lot of changes in medicine and surgery. It was because of all the dreadful injuries caused to soldiers in the trenches during the First World War (1914–1918) that Alexander Flemming tried to look for an antibiotic drug to combat blood poisoning (see chapter 32). It took a long time to develop the drug, but **E** shows Flemming's view of its worth during the Second World War (1939–45).

❛*The first man I tried it on was a young New Zealand officer. He had been in bed for six months with compound fractures in both legs. His sheets were saturated with pus. He was little more than skin and bone and was running a high temperature. Normally he would have died in a very short while. We injected him with a very weak solution of penicillin. Out there in Cairo, I knew nothing of what was being done in England and the thing seemed like a miracle. In ten days the first leg was cured and in a month the fellow was back on his feet.*❜ (**E**)

??????????????????

1 a If the only evidence you had about the development of surgery were the pictures **A** and **D**, what conclusions would you come to about the effect of war on the progress of surgical techniques?

b What does your answer to **a** teach you about the value of photographs as historical evidence?

2 Look at **B**, **C** and **E** and in each case describe how they show an example of how war has accelerated progress in medicine.

3 In what ways do you think war slowed down progress in medicine?

4 What similarities are there between what Pare did (**B**) and Pulverstaff (the doctor who wrote **E**) did?

5 Write or tape a debate between two people, one who thinks that, on the whole, war had a good effect on the development of medicine and another who thinks that, on the whole, it had a bad effect.

39 Religious Belief and Medicine

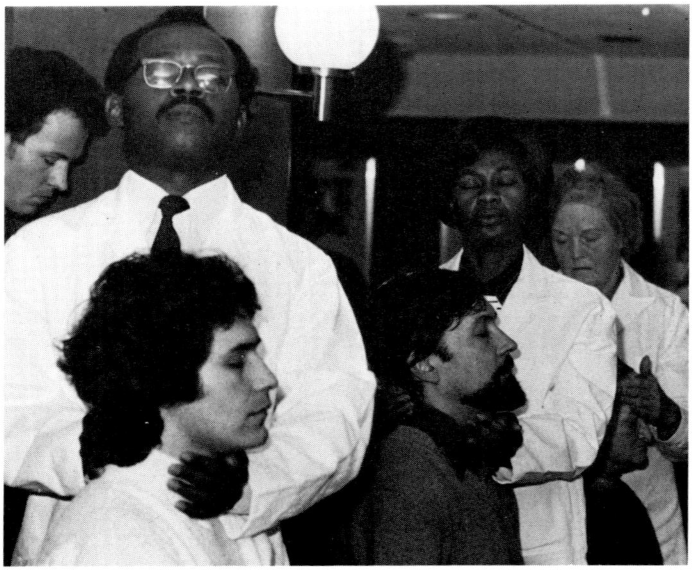

A A group of faith healers in action

A shows a group of faith healers in action. Many people find that they can be cured of illnesses by having faith in the healing powers of someone. Religious belief involves people trusting their god to guide them. They can't see or touch their god, nor prove that their god exists; but they believe in its power.

Such belief can both speed up and slow down progress. Look at the Red Indian medicine man (**B**). The Indian tribes believed that these medicine men had been given special powers to heal the sick. Do you think this belief would have accelerated or slowed down progress in medical knowledge among the North American Indians?

Religious belief has been both a driving force for change in medicine (*an agent of change*) and a barrier against change (*an inhibitor of change*).

Religious belief as an inhibitor of change

Earlier in this book you learnt that their religion forbade the Ancient Egyptians to dissect human bodies because it was believed the spirit of a dead person would need the body in their after–life. This prevented the Egyptians learning about some internal organs of the body. You will also remember that the Greeks often trusted in gods such as Asclepios (see chapter 4) to cure their illnesses; this hardly encouraged growth in knowledge about medicine.

Up until the 13th century, the Christian Church discouraged dissection of the human body and the following comment by St Bernard in the 12th century shows that the church did not wholeheartedly support investigation into medical research:

‘*To buy drugs or consult with physicians doesn't fit with religion.*’ (**C**)

As late as the 1660s in England, many people still believed that a religious figure could cure their illnesses for them. One major disease was known as *Scrofula*. The people believed that the King was God's representative on earth and the following extract shows how they thought the King could cure their disease:

‘*The sick are brought or led up to the throne where they kneel; the King strokes their faces or cheeks with both hands at once, at which instance a chaplain in his formality says "He put his hands upon them and healed them".*’ (**D**)

From John Evlyn's diary, 1660

B A red indian medicine man

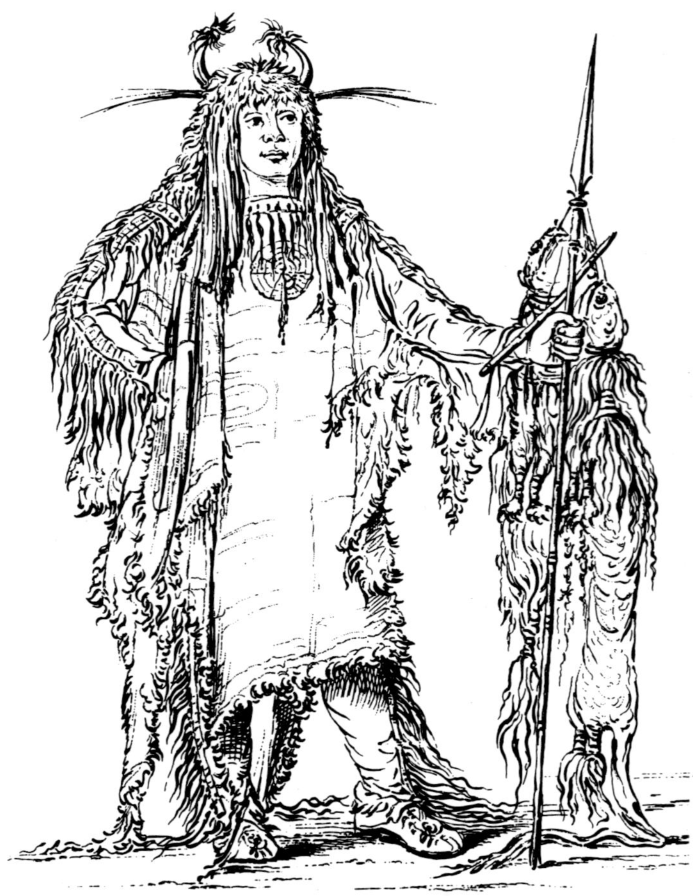

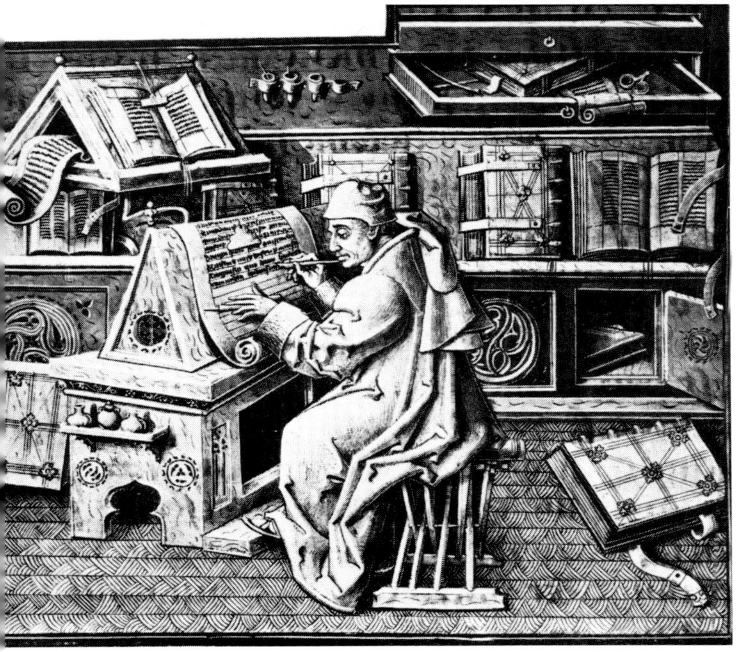

E A monk translating books

Religious belief as an agent of change

Religious beliefs and practices have also encouraged or speeded up progress in medicine. They have often been an *agent of change* in medicine. You have already seen in chapter 13 that the monks in the Middle Ages learnt about the value of hygiene as part of their religion, and how monasteries became the major centres for the treatment of the sick during those times. Perhaps more important still was the work of monks like the one in **E**.

People such as the monk in **E** translated important medical books into Latin. Latin was a language that scholars from many different countries could read. Many important medical books such as Galen's work (see chapter 8) were translated into Latin and this kept alive some of the better ideas about medical practice.

From the 12th century onwards the church took a more active role in education and helped to set up more than 1,200 universities throughout Europe such as the famous medical school at Salerno (see chapter 10). It was from universities such as these that many of the developments in medicine during the Renaissance (1500–1700) came.

Just as we saw earlier that blind faith or trust in something can prevent people from bothering to learn things for themselves, many religious people would argue that their belief in religion has given them a motive or a reason to investigate into medicine, so that they can use their knowledge to help others. Dr Christian Barnard (see chapter 33) is a good example of such a person. **E** shows what he wrote about the first heart transplant operation that he performed in 1967.

'I always pray before any major operation ... And then, as I drove through the night, I felt more than ever the need to pray ... Each time I began my thoughts broke in on me. Dear Lord, help me with this operation.' (**E**)
(One Life *by Christian Barnard Harrap and Co. Ltd., 1969).*

?????????????????

1 Complete a chart like the one below. Yours will need to be drawn bigger in order to fit all the information in.

(i) Source (describe)	**(ii) Primary/ Secondary**	**(iii) Agent/ Inhibitor of change**	**(iv) Detail to support (iii)**
A Picture of a faith healer	Primary	Inhibitor	People should try to find scientific solutions to illnesses.
B Medicine man			
C St Bernard's opinion			
D Charles II touching someone			
E A monk writing			
F A surgeon praying			

2 Using this chapter, and your knowledge from the rest of this book, make two lists:

i Ways in which religious belief has helped progress in medicine.
ii Ways in which religious belief has hindered progress in medicine.

3 Look back over chapters 36–38. Which of the following do you think has had the greatest effect on the progress of medicine: war, technology, or religious belief? Make sure you write about each one, giving examples, before reaching your conclusion.

40 Modern Day Living and Health Problems

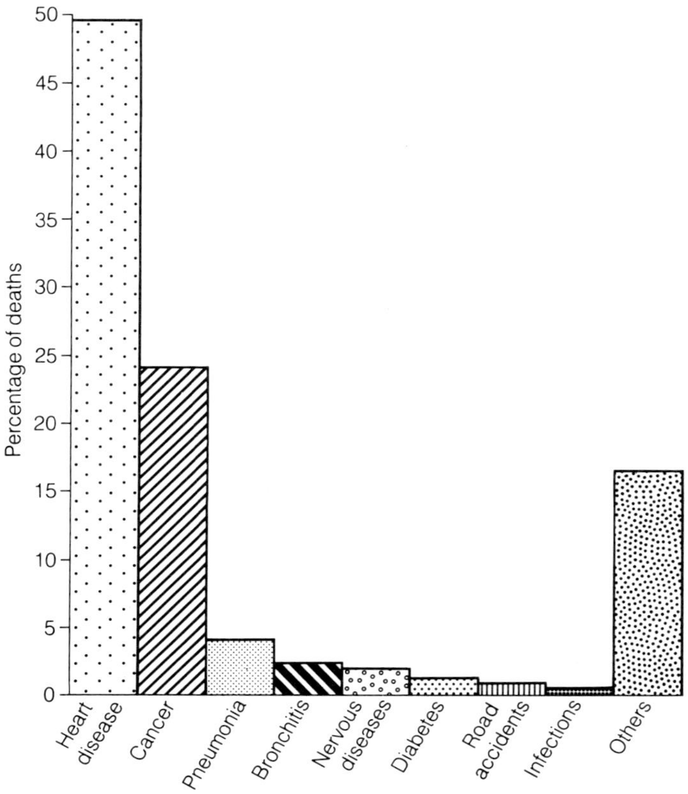

A Causes of death in Britain in the 1980s

Take a look around your class. There are probably about thirty of you. If you had been alive 150 years ago, you could only have expected to live, on average, to the age of 40. Today, you are more likely to live to 70 or more. The main causes of death 150 years ago were Measles, Cholera, Typhoid and Diptheria, all of which can now be cured or prevented quite easily. We all have to die eventually of course, but today the main causes of death are different (**A**) and some of them are brought about by the way we live.

Of the people in your class, 14 are likely to die of heart disease, seven from cancer, one or two from pneumonia and the rest from the other causes shown on the graph.

We don't yet know exactly what causes cancer, but we have got some very good ideas about how to prevent heart disease, Britain's major killer. Doctors strongly believe that we should all exercise for twenty-minute periods, three times a week. Vigorous exercise raises the pulse rate and helps the heart muscles to develop and become stronger and more able to fight disease. Other things to do to avoid heart disease include being careful about your weight by trying to stay slim (but equally you must be careful not to diet unnecessarily as this can be dangerous). We should avoid eating fatty foods such as chips or fried meats, and leave sugar out of our drinks. We should also try to eat wholemeal bread and plenty of fruit and vegetables. All this should help us to live longer, and enjoy life more fully at the same time.

Stress is a 'modern day' disease. Overwork and anxiety about such things as bills, causes thousands of people to be nervous or fidgety, over-anxious and depressed. Hundreds of thousands of workdays are lost each year because of stress.

Many people believe cigarettes to be the other major cause of death today. Smoking is said to cause cancer and

B An anti-smoking poster

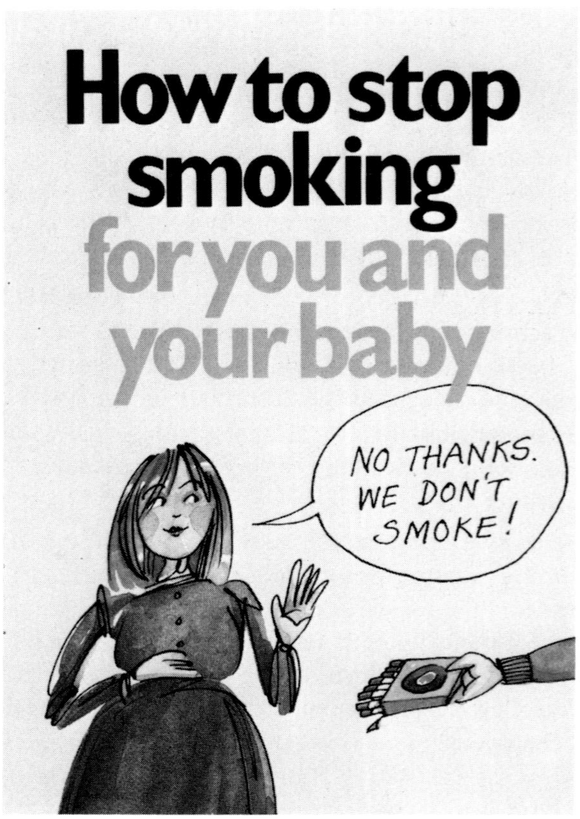

How to stop smoking
for you and your baby
NO THANKS. WE DON'T SMOKE!

bronchitis. Many of us are in danger from *passive smoking*, by breathing in the cigarette smoke of someone else, even if we don't smoke. Women who smoke during pregnancy are more likely to have small or deformed babies (**B**). Smoking is considered to be such a major health risk that many measures have been taken against smokers: there are 'no smoking' areas in many public places such as cinemas or restaurants and the advertising of cigarettes on television is banned. All other advertisements for cigarettes carry the Government Health Warning: 'Cigarettes can seriously damage your health'.

C An AIDS information leaflet

HOW MANY PEOPLE ARE AFFECTED?

By the end of September 1987 it was estimated that about 50,000 people in the UK had been infected with HIV. 1,067 of these had developed AIDS.

In the UK, 84% of people with AIDS are homosexual or bisexual men. But in a number of African countries, for example, AIDS affects men and women equally. No-one knows for sure why AIDS has followed such a different pattern there.

Worldwide, 60,653 cases had been reported to the World Health Organisation from 152 countries by the end of September 1987. Of these, 41,825 were in the United States.

Cases of AIDS in the UK up to the end of September 1987:

901 **Homosexual or bisexual men**
Homosexuals are men who have sexual intercourse with other men. Bisexual men have sexual intercourse with women and men.

83 **Haemophiliacs and people who were infected by blood transfusion**
Haemophiliacs are people who repeatedly need special blood products to help their blood to clot. Since 1985 in this country, all donated blood has been screened for antibodies to HIV, and blood products heat treated. This has greatly reduced the risk of people getting the virus in this way.

32 **Drug misusers**
Those who inject themselves.

51 **Others**
These include men and women who seem to have caught the virus by having sex with an infected partner of the opposite sex, and children of mothers infected with HIV.

Total = 1,067 By October 1987, 605 of these people had died of AIDS.

Source **C**, however, discusses what is probably the fastest growing disease today. When this book was first published in 1984, virtually no one had heard of it. Now, many doctors consider that it will soon be one of the major causes of death in Britain.

AIDS stands for 'Acquired Immune Deficiency Syndrome' and it is a disease that prevents the body from fighting off other illnesses that normally it could cope with quite easily. At the time of writing, there is no known cure for the disease.

But we must not think that modern day living is all bad news. Many of the diseases or causes of illness mentioned in this chapter have, after all, only come to our attention because doctors have managed to cure many of the major illnesses and diseases that used to cause death over a hundred years ago. A hundred years ago, most people didn't live long enough to die of things such as lung cancer or heart failure. Modern advances in surgery, treatment and drugs have made the world, in general, a healthier place to live. Many of the illnesses mentioned above occur because people don't look after themselves as well as they should.

??????????????????

1 i Why do people tend to live longer now than they did 150 years ago?
ii The fact that people live longer these days means that more than a third of Britain's population are now over the age of sixty. Make a list of the problems this can cause for doctors and for society as a whole.

2 In what ways could it be said that 'modern day living' styles can make people unhealthy?

3 Using **C**, compile a list of the people most likely to catch Aids. Write a leaflet or design a poster that would appeal to your own age group warning people how to avoid catching the disease.

4 Using all the evidence in this chapter, compile a list of all the things people should do to stay healthy. Carry out a survey in your class and compile a graph of the results. Then comment on how healthy/unhealthy you think your class is.

41 Progress and change

The next two chapters should be studied together. They are about why things happen in history and the effects of historical events. This chapter deals with the *causes* of historical events and the next chapter deals with the *effects* and with the pace or speed of change. In a book called 'What Is History', the historian E H Carr gives an example of a person who runs out of cigarettes. They are killed by a car while crossing the road to buy another packet of cigarettes. What was the cause of their death?

Effectively, there were many causes, some of them *long term causes* (things that happened a long time before the event) and some of them were *short term causes* (things that happened much closer to the event). There are many causes that go together to make something happen (**A**). Sometimes the long term causes are more important and sometimes it is the short term ones. In Carr's example you *could* say that the smoker was killed because they smoked; because if they hadn't smoked they probably wouldn't have crossed the road to buy a packet of cigarettes at that precise moment. Similarly, they probably wouldn't have been killed if the motor car engine had not been invented so the invention of the motor car could be said to be a cause of death!

In any historical event, it is the job of the historian to try to work out all the possible causes and then try to decide which were the most important ones. It is rare that an event only has one cause. It is usually a combination of many of the types of causes shown in **A**.

Let's look at an example from this book. In Chapter 18 you read about Louis Pasteur. Louis Pasteur was the man who realised that microbes caused disease. He discovered this because he was asked by the French wine industry to

A Why things happen in history

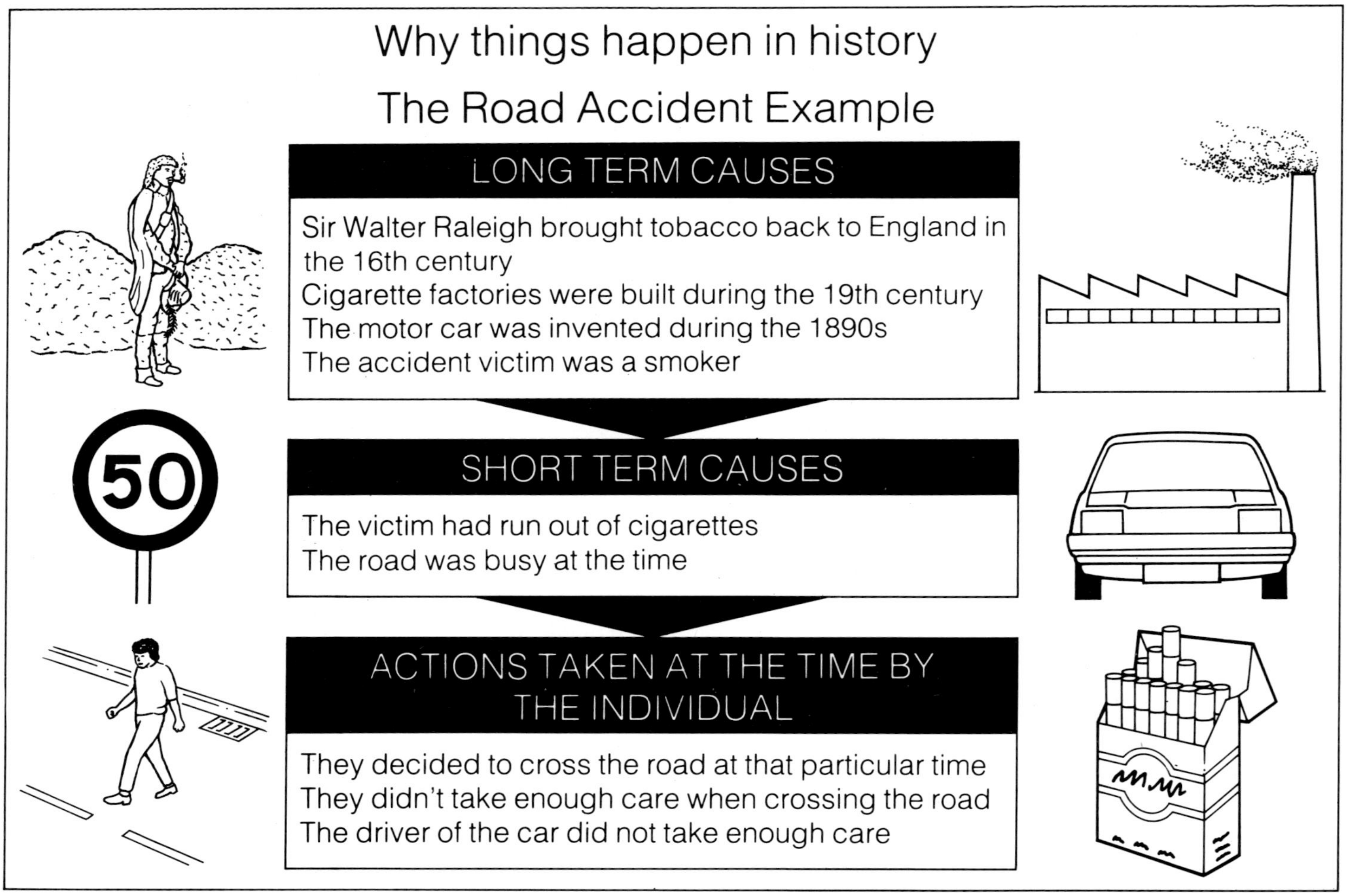

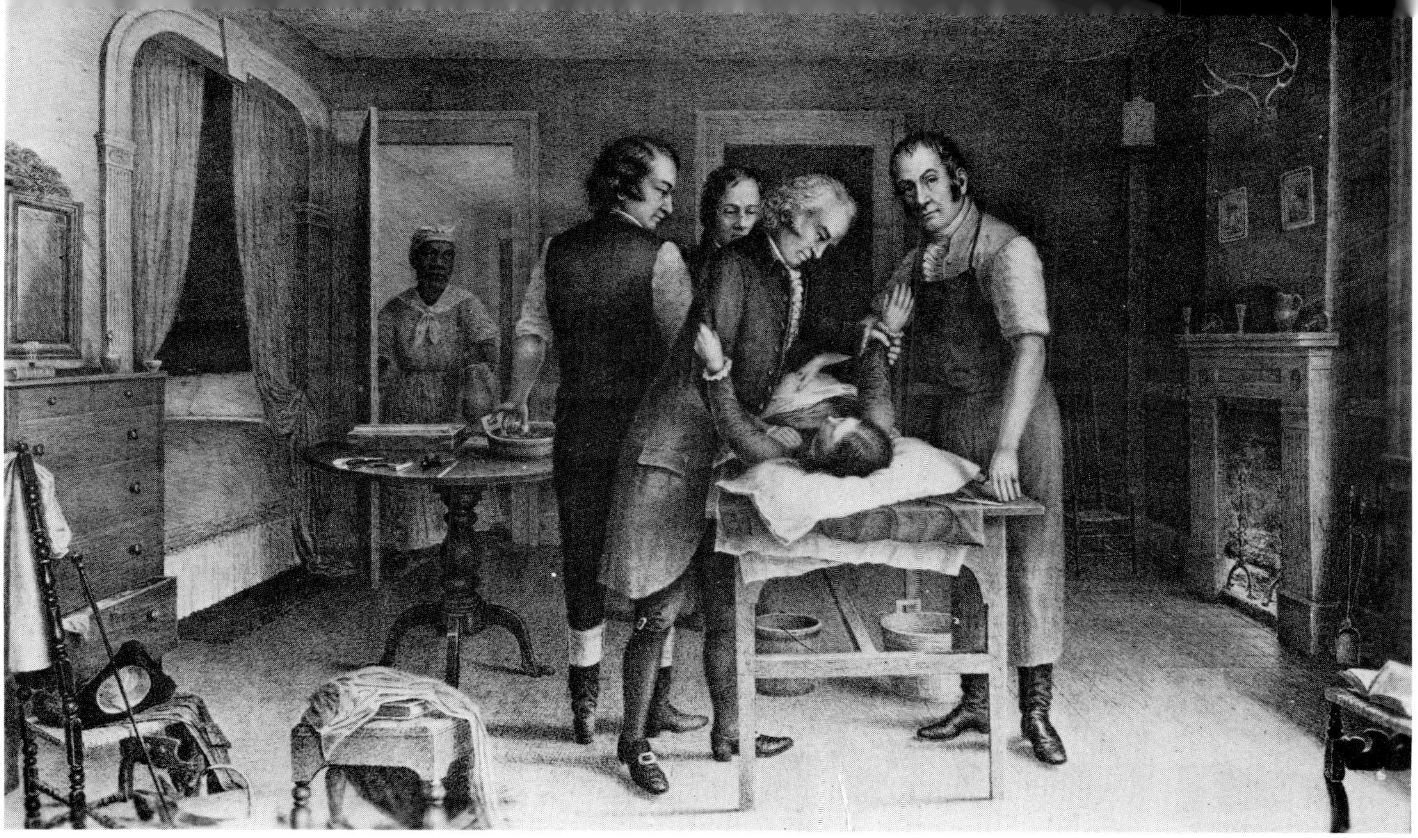

B This drawing recreates an operation in 1809 where a woman had her ovaries removed without anaesthetic

investigate why wine sometimes went sour. By experimentation he saw that it was only when air got into the wine that it went sour and, later, he managed to see the bacteria, that were causing the problem, under a microscope.

If you were answering the question 'How and why did Louis Pasteur discover the existence of bacteria?' you would have to include *long term causes* such as the discovery of the microscope and the idea of scientific experimentation, that were used by Pasteur. You would have to mention the more immediate or *short term causes* such as the fact he was asked to look at the problem by the French wine industry. You would have to include actions taken by Pasteur himself; for instance, the decision he made to boil the liquid and seal it, keeping it away from air. It is then a case of deciding which were the most important causes and reaching a conclusion.

Another major debate in history is whether the individual or the actions taken by individuals are historically more important than the circumstances. To make this idea a bit easier to understand, look at **B** which shows a picture of a woman having her ovaries removed (without anaesthetic) in 1809. The surgeons in this example are obviously learning a great deal about gynaecology (see chapter 23) and so the actions that they, as individuals, are taking are very important. You might say that their actions are bringing about change. But it can also be argued that the place and time they were in, allowed them to carry out this work and so the *circumstances* were more important. If these men had lived in an Islamic country, for instance, where men were not allowed to practice gynaecology, they wouldn't have been able to carry out the operation.

????????????????????

1 Redraw diagram **A** or ask your teacher to produce some blank outlines of it. Put in just the main headings in each box: *Long term causes*, *Short term causes*, and *Actions taken by the individual*. Fill in the gaps for each of the following events you have studied in this book: the discovery of clinical observation by Hippocrates; William Harvey's discovery of the circulation of the blood; Edward Jenner's discovery of vaccination; Joseph Lister's discovery of antiseptics.

2 Which do you think were the most important causes of these discoveries: the long term, the short term, the actions of the individual, or a combination of all three. Explain your answer.

3 Highlight some actions taken by individuals in the examples you have studied for question **1**. Say why you think these individual actions were important.

42 The most important events

In the last chapter you learnt about what causes certain historical events to happen. In this chapter we will concentrate on the *effects* (consequences) of historical events in order to try to discover whether some events in the history of medicine have been more important than others. In order to understand this idea more clearly, here is an activity for the whole class to do.

Historical consequences game

Many of you will have played the game *Consequences* where someone writes a boy's name on a piece of paper, folds it over and passes it to the next person who writes a girl's name on it, and so on. Historical consequences is a similar game but it helps you to understand how events can have different consequences depending on the conditions at the time that they happen.

Your teacher will divide you into groups of four or five. He or she will then write an event from this book on the top of a piece of paper and give it to the first person in your group. (The event might be something like 'The microscope was invented' or 'William Harvey discovered the circulation of the blood'.)

The first person in the group must write down what the immediate consequences or effects of the event would have been and then fold over the paper so that the next person can only see what they have just written, *not* the event at the top of the page. The process is repeated until everyone in the group has written something. The teacher will then summarise each group's consequences on the board. Then see if you can answer these questions about your class results.

1 Were the final or last consequences generally good or bad?

2 Were the final consequences what they really turned out to be or were they different from what really happened?

3 If they were different, then why was this so? What things didn't happen in reality that people thought might happen when they wrote them down as consequences?

4 What does all the above tell you about change and the reasons why things change in history.

5 Now look at the three pictures, **A**, **B** and **C**. You have seen them all earlier in this book. Write a few sentences explaining how **A** helped lead to **B** and how the two of them helped lead to **C**.

What you have been doing in the exercises above is making links between things that happened many years apart. This will help you to see how things and events in history have an effect on each other but also that one thing on its own does not lead to another. It takes many causes to make up an event and the consequences or effects of an event can be different depending on the circumstances.

For instance, if somebody tries to invent something or discovers something and the situation isn't quite right for other people to see the value of that discovery, then the chances of that discovery having any great effect are very small. For instance, Franz Gall (1758–1828) tried to convince people that different parts of the brain controlled different parts of a person's character and that you could tell what sort of person they would turn out to be in later life by feeling bumps along certain parts of the head near the brain. Brain surgery was an impossibility at the time because the necessary technology had not been developed and Gall's ideas didn't come to anything. However, it is now largely recognised that his theories were in many ways correct since more research on the brain has been possible.

There are many more examples like this. It helps to make it clearer if we think of the many recent medical discoveries that would have been ridiculed if they had been suggested, say, 200 years ago because the circumstances were not just right for people to accept them (the idea of test-tube babies for instance or of antiseptic surgery).

Further questions

6 Find examples from this book to prove or disprove each of the following statements:
'Progress brings good results'; 'Progress brings bad results'; 'Some changes happen very quickly'; 'Some changes take hundreds of years to come about'; 'People are healthier now than they were 200 years ago'.

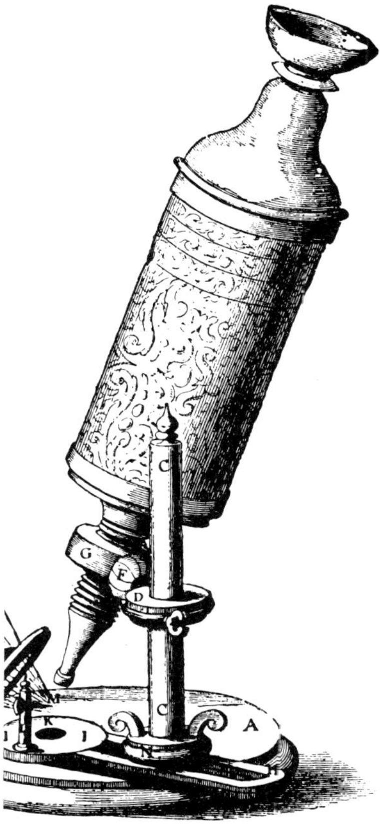

A Microscope made by the Englishman Robert Hooke in 1665

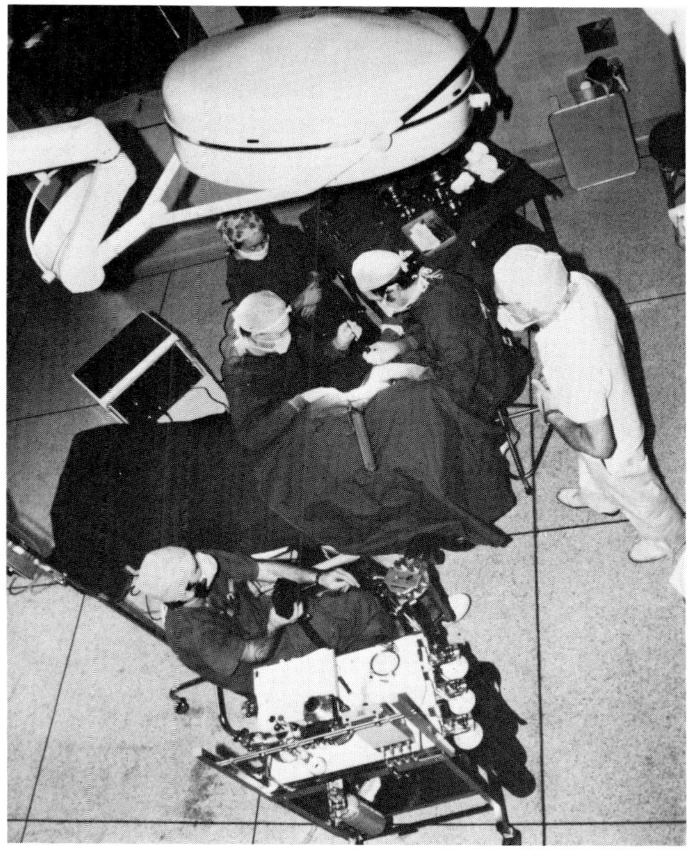

C A modern operating theatre

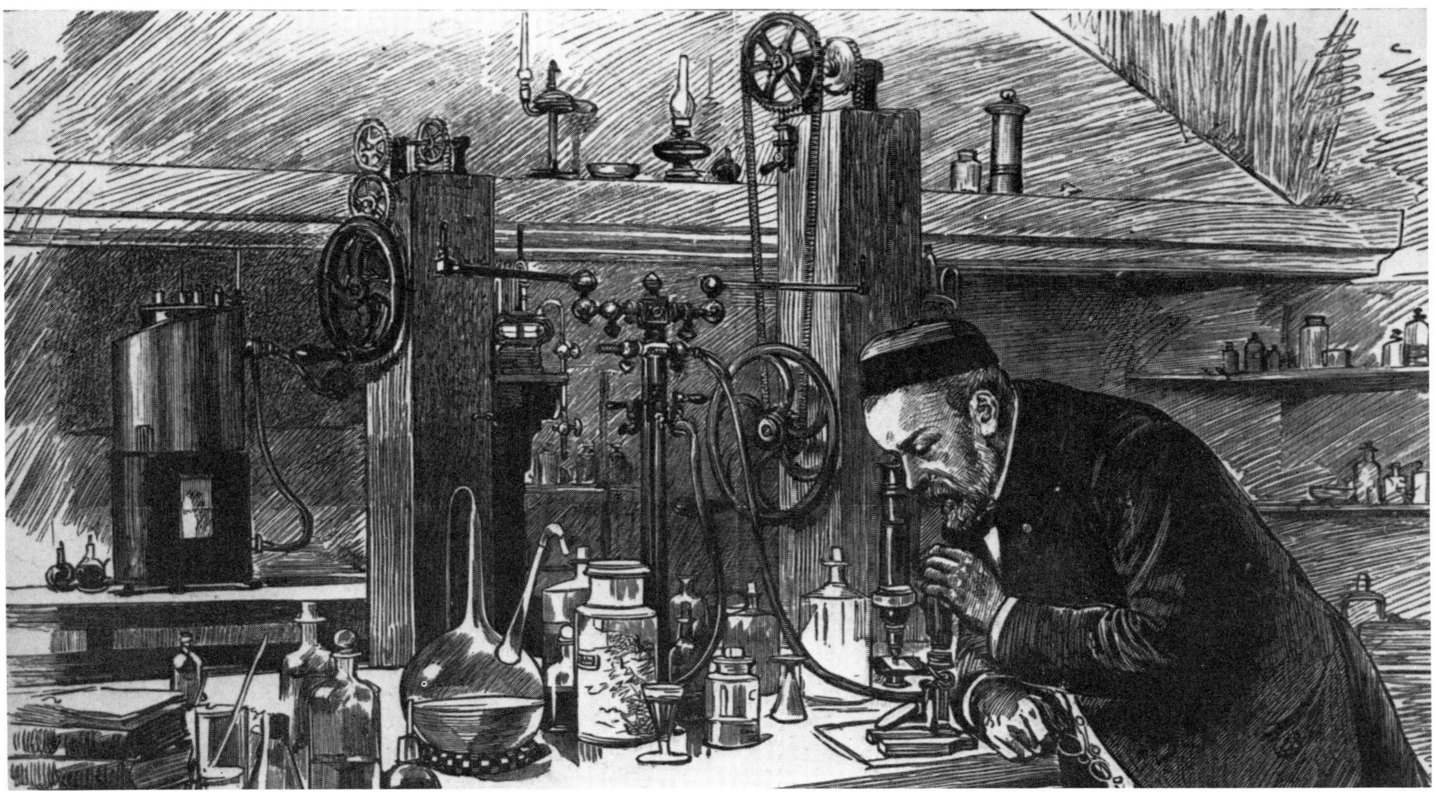

B Pasteur in his laboratory

43 The Revision Game

Instructions

Split the form up into two teams. Each member of each team can ask an opposing member of the other team *one* question. If the answer is correct, that team gains one mark. If the question is not answered, or the wrong answer is given, the team asking the question gains one mark.

Teams take it in turn to ask one question at a time.

QUESTIONS

Prehistoric Times

What was the name of the operation where holes were drilled in skulls? 1
Name a religious belief held by early man. 1
Name a superstitious belief held by early man. 1
Name one way early man kept healthy. 1
Give the rough dates of the Babylonian Empire. 6
In what way did the Babylonians forecast disease? 6
Who wrote a code of laws in 1930 BC? 6

Egyptian Times

What are the rough dates of the ancient Egyptians? 2
What was embalming? 2
Who became the Egyptian god of healing? 2
Name a religious belief of the ancient Egyptians. 2
Name a superstitious belief of the ancient Egyptians. 2
Who was Edwin Smith? 2
What was papyrus? 2
Name one organ of the body the Egyptians studied. 2
Name one way the Egyptians were hygienic. 2
How did a settled way of life in Egyptian times help the development of medicine? 2
Why couldn't the Egyptians dissect the human body? 2
Name a medical cure from Egyptian times. 2

Ancient Greece

Name a magical cure the Greeks believed in. 3
Name a famous Greek Doctor. 3
Name one way the Greeks kept fit. 3
How did trade help the development of medicine in Greece? 3
Name a Greek philosopher. 3
What did Plato and Aristotle prove? 3
What was at Alexandria? 3
What did Erasistratus prove? 3
What were Asclepaeia? 4
What was in the entrance hall to an Asclepaeia? 4
Name two of the four humours. 5
Name a piece of advice that Hippocrates gave. 5
What is the Hippocratic Oath? 5

The Romans

Who carried first aid kits? 7
Name the country where military hospitals have been found. 7
Name one way the Romans kept healthy. 7
What were aqueducts? 7
What was the entrance fee to the Baths? 7
Name a piece of advice concerning health given to Roman soldiers. 7
What was the Cloaca Maxima? 7
Why didn't the Romans like doctors 7
Name two of the rooms you would find in a Roman bath. 7
Name a famous Roman surgeon. 8
State one way Galen was wrong. 8
How did gladiators help Galen? 8
What nationality was Galen? 8

The Dark Ages

Why are they called the Dark Ages? 9
Roughly what dates were the Dark Ages? 9
Why did the Roman Empire fall? 9
Name a nonsensical remedy in the Dark Ages. 9
Name a place where medicine was kept alive. 9
Name an Arab centre of learning. 10
Who was Nestorius? 10
Name a famous Arab doctor. 11
What did Albicasis do? 11

The Middle Ages

What was the zodiac chart? 12
What animals did surgeons dissect? (Name two) 12
What was bloodletting? 12
How did the church inhibit change in medicine? 12
What was the remedy for toothache? 12
What other jobs did surgeons have? 12
What was a vademecum? 12
Name one way monasteries were hygienic. 13
What date was the Black Death in England? 13
Name something people thought would cure the Black Death. 13
What did people use as soap? 13
Who were Flagellants? 13
How were lepers treated? 13

The Renaissance

Give the rough dates of the Renaissance. 14
How did artists help in the development of medicine? 14
How did the printing press help in the development of medicine? 14
How did discoverers help the development of medicine? 14
Name one thing Paracelsus did. 14
Name one thing Thomas Sydenham did. 14
Which university had a famous anatomical theatre? 14
What did Paré do? 15
What did Harvey discover? 15
How did warfare help the development of surgery? 15
What nationality was Harvey? 15
Name the book written by Vesalius. 15
Name the book written by Paré. 15
Name the book written by Harvey. 15

First published in 1984 by Basil Blackwell Limited
Reprinted in 1984, 1985, 1986, 1989

Second edition published in 1992 by Simon & Schuster Education
Reprinted 1992, 1993

Reprinted in 1994 by Stanley Thornes (Publishers) Ltd
Ellenborough House
Wellington Street
CHELTENHAM GL50 1YD
England

A catalogue record for this book is available from the British Library.

ISBN 0 7487 1957 1

Printed in Hong Kong by Wing King Tong Co. Ltd.

Acknowledgements

Ann Ronan Picture Library 13(F), 19(A), 22(B), 27(C), 30(B), 37(D), 40(C), 45(E), 48(B), 51(B), 53(E); Ashmolean Museum, Oxford 4(B), 6(A), 7(C); British Museum 18(B); BBC Hulton Picture Library 23(D), 33(D), 36(B), 38(C), 44(B), 47(B,E), 60(C), 36(B,C), 37(B), 39(A,B,E), 41(B), 42(B); Complutense University of Madrid (Faculty of Medicine); Daily Telegraph 41(F); Deutsches Archaeologisches Institut 10(B); Health Education Authority 40(B); International General Electric Company of New York 58(B); IWM 38(D); John Watney Photo Library 39(F), 59(C), 61(D); Mansell Collection 2(A), 5(C), 8(C), 9(Da,b), 12(B), 14(A,D), 16(A), 21(E) and cover, 24(A), 31(A), 35(D), 40(B), 43(E), 49(D); Mary Evans Picture Library 42(A); Museum of London 29(F); Papworth Hospital Heart Transplant Unit 59(E); Pitt Rivers Museum 5(D); Popperfoto 10(A), 56(B); Science Museum 2(B), 3(C,D), 4(A), 13(D), 18(A), 20(D), 27(E), 34(A), 37(F), 39(D), 50(C), 56(A), 57(D); Sonia Halliday Photographs 6(B); John Watney 42(C); Jon Vogler 35(A); Wayland Picture Library 25(D), 26(A), 27(F), 34(B), 58(A); Weidenfeld and Nicholson Picture Archive 8(A); Wellcome Institute Library, London 11(C), 23(G), 24(B); Who (E. Schwab) 35(C); World Health Organisation 55(C,E).

Index